Orem's Model in Action

STEPHEN J. CAVANAGH

RGN, BA(Nurs.), MS, MPA, Ph.D., MBIM
Division of Nursing,
School of Health Sciences,
Wolverhampton Polytechnic

Series Editor

BOB PRICE

BA, M.Sc., SRN, Cert.Ed.(Education)
Army Medical Services School of Nursing,
Woolwich

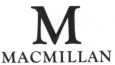

MACMILLAN

To
Lindy, Andrew and Ben

First published 1991 by
THE MACMILLAN PRESS LTD
Houndmills, Basingstoke, Hampshire RG21 2XS
and London
Companies and representatives
throughout the world

Designed by Claire Brodmann

ISBN 0–333–53624–X

A catalogue record for this book is available
from the British Library.

Printed in China

Reprinted 1992 (twice), 1993

CONTENTS

Certain conventions have been observed in the writing of this book. First, a person receiving nursing care is usually referred to as a 'patient', but in some contexts as a 'client'; the terms are often interchangeable and their use tends to be dictated by local practice. Secondly, people in the book are usually referred to by their first name only – this reflects the trust established in effective nurse–patient relationships; each patient is understood to have consented to this use of his or her name. Thirdly, unless the context requires otherwise the nurse is referred to as 'she' and the patient as 'he'. These conventions are solely for reasons of simplicity, clarity and style.

Of all the nursing care models that have evolved within the USA, Dorothea Orem's has been perhaps the most influential. Adopted widely within the UK, Europe and elsewhere, it has offered a refreshingly direct approach to modern care situations. The notions of 'self-care' and of nurses making very active decisions on just how much to intervene with patients – choosing a 'nursing care system' – appeal to the profession today. The economics of health care, and a rising tide of health-care consumerism, mean that nurses must consider carefully just what role they should play with a patient. Often to intervene strongly, to act *for* patients, is inappropriate, undermining their motivation to look after themselves when they have the capacity to do so. This may be not only an untherapeutic approach but one that invades personal privacy and threatens the individual's dignity. Some nursing care may best be presented in the form of education and support, teaching or guiding the patient in self-care measures.

On ethical, legal and professional grounds, nurses must now carefully reflect on the care they plan, deliver and eventually evaluate. The Orem model facilitates this effectively, addressing the patient's self-care deficits through a wide-ranging assessment. The model covers not only universal self-care need (self-care requisites), but also those needs specific to the individual's physical, social and psychological development, and to this encounter with illness or injury and with the caring professions (developmental and health-deviation self-care requisites).

Having accepted that Orem's work is of major importance to nursing, we are still faced with a need to examine her concepts of care in action. This is particularly important when such concepts must be taken out of the context of American culture and clinical nursing practice and transplanted into nursing-care settings within the UK and elsewhere. In short, we need to draw upon informed interpretation of the model, and to this end Stephen Cavanagh's volume will be most welcome. Personal contact with Orem-based care in the USA, and an established reputation for teaching the model's concepts to nurses, equips him to help the reader deal with the exciting new ideas and perspectives that Orem offers.

Once the nurse has moved beyond the difficulty of wrestling with new concepts and 'foreign semantics', the Orem model of care can seem delightfully simple. In many respects this is as it should be, given that it is designed for practical use by nurses in busy clinical settings. Nevertheless, it should not be underestimated as a piece of nursing theory, for the nurse who really practises Orem-based care can no longer rely on ritualised practice or avoid partnering the patient in very active care-planning. Orem-based nursing care involves the nurse in some honest decisions and a fundamental rethink of the caring relationship. To this end, the care studies in Part II, and the balanced critique of the model in Part III, will be invaluable.

This then is a volume intended to be of interest to nurses, student and qualified alike. It is eminently practical, explaining the model in the context of varied examples of patient situations, but never accepting its tenets without healthy criticism. It is a volume that joins the many on nursing models, but it stands out as an informed interpretation, and one by which I am sure nurses will feel encouraged.

Bob Price

PART I

Orem's model today

CHAPTER ONE

The meaning of nursing

INTRODUCTION

Dorothea Orem's model of nursing has found increasing popularity worldwide as a means of organising the knowledge, the skills and the motivation of nurses that are needed to deliver care to patients. As with other nursing models, the practical application and conceptual underpinning of Orem's work has generally not been fully discussed in the United Kingdom – in fact, the model has tended to be viewed as synonymous with the concept of self-care, which actually constitutes only one part of the model, and not necessarily the most important one. This chapter discusses a wide range of issues emerging from Orem's work, and culminates with practical ways of using the model to assess, plan, deliver and evaluate patient care.

The language of the model

There has been much discussion in the literature complaining that many models originating in the United States are complicated, unworkable and unintelligible. A principal aspect criticised has been the language used. This is unfortunate because the task of describing nursing roles and functions does sometimes require specifically defined terms that are clear and unambiguous; constructing these terms has been difficult. The failure of many American theorists is not in their use of specialised terms (so-called jargon) but in their failure to communicate what they mean in a way that is understandable. This chapter introduces some of the key terms in Orem's language in a way that aims to ensure that the model does make sense. You may contest Orem's perspectives – that is all part of the analytical and critical nature of education – but you must have a clear basis for your opinions. Understanding the language of the model is the first step in making well-reasoned judgements.

The origins of the model

Dorothea Orem's quest for a greater understanding of the nature of nursing formally began in the late 1950s, and focused on three questions:

1 What *do* nurses do, and what *should* nurses do, as practitioners of nursing?
2 *Why* do nurses do what they do?
3 What are the results of nursing interventions?

(adapted from Orem and Taylor 1986, p.37)

The desire to address these issues emerged from substantial practical experience, including work as a staff nurse in medicine, surgery and paediatrics, and as a casualty and theatre sister. During time spent teaching biological sciences and nursing, as well as being a director of a hospital school of nursing, Orem dedicated much energy to understanding the meaning of nursing. The current formulation of her work, *Nursing: Concepts of Practice* (1991), has undergone substantial revision since earlier work appeared in 1971, 1980 and 1985. Such revisions have been based upon comments and discussion raised at nursing theory conferences but also on the reactions of the people using the model. Orem does not claim that her model is by any means the complete answer to her questions or a panacea for practice. She simply provides a framework in which to view nursing practice, education and management. It is for each individual practitioner to use this model for its intended purpose: to improve nursing care.

THE NATURE OF SELF-CARE

At its simplest, *self-care* could be considered to be the ability of an individual to manage all the activities needed to live and survive. Orem views 'self' as the totality of an individual, including not only his physical but also his psychological and spiritual needs, and 'care' as the totality of activities that an individual initiates to maintain life and to develop in a way that is normal for himself. Self-care is the practice of activities that individuals initiate and perform on their own behalf in maintaining life, health and well-being (Orem 1991, p.117). Specifically, an individual can be considered to be self-caring if the following are effectively managed:

- support of life processes and normal functioning;
- maintenance of normal growth, maturation and development;
- prevention or control of disease processes and injuries;
- prevention of, or compensation for, disability;
- promotion of well-being.

Central to the concept of self-care is that care is being initiated voluntarily and deliberately by an individual. People may not spend much time thinking about the specific actions they take to maintain their health or natural development; day-to-day living can become an automatic process. Self-care, however, should not be considered as a set of routine actions that individuals perform without thinking or making decisions: quite the contrary is true, in fact, for self-care is an active phenomenon requiring people to be able to use reason to understand their health condition, and decision-making skills to choose an appropriate course of action. In this sense self-care is the practice, after consideration, of activities that will maintain life and health and also promote well-being. The activities necessary to maintain health and development are learned, and are influenced by many factors including age, maturation and culture.

Assumptions about the nature of man

In order to understand, use and criticise Orem's model, it is important to consider some of the assumptions she makes about the nature of human beings:

1 All things being equal, human beings have the potential to develop intellectual and practical skills and to maintain the motivation essential for self-care and care for dependent family members. This places the responsibility on the individuals, wherever possible, to manage their own care needs by developing the necessary information and skills, or by finding assistance from other sources such as relatives or professional practitioners including nurses.

2 Ways of meeting self-care requisites are cultural elements and vary with individuals and with larger social groups. The definition of when help from others is needed, and the specific actions used to meet their needs, will vary according to the societal or cultural group to which the individual belongs. This suggests that there is no 'one way' to meet the demands of self-care; instead, different approaches can be used to meet similar needs.

3 The performance of self-care requires deliberate, calculated action which is influenced by an individual's knowledge and skills repertoire, and which is based upon the premise that individuals know when they are in need of assistance and are aware of the specific actions they therefore need to take. Individuals do, however, have choices in self-caring behaviour. In certain circumstances an individual may decide, for whatever reason, not to initiate self-care behaviours when they are needed. Reasons include anxiety, fear, or other priorities.

4 Individuals will investigate and develop ways to meet known self-care demands. When faced with the realisation of having self-care needs, they will experiment and try different methods to overcome their difficulties. When ways to meet known needs are identified, they will develop self-care habits.

(adapted from Orem 1991, p.69)

SELF-CARE REQUISITES

Essential to Orem's model are so-called *self-care requisites*. Not only are these a major component of the model, but they also form an important part of patient assessment (discussed later in this chapter). Orem (1991, p.121) has identified and described eight activities that are essential to the attainment of self-care, irrespective of an individual's health status, age, level of development or environmental surroundings. These activities are called *universal self-care requisites*. The term 'requisite' is used to mean an activity that an individual must perform in order to be self-caring. There are two further kinds of self-care requisite, *developmental* and *health-care deviation requisites*, which will be discussed later.

Universal self-care requisites

The eight self-care requisites common to all human beings include:

1 the maintenance of a sufficient intake of air;
2 the maintenance of a sufficient intake of water;
3 the maintenance of a sufficient intake of food;
4 the provision of care associated with elimination processes and excrements;
5 the maintenance of a balance between activity and rest;
6 the maintenance of a balance between solitude and social integration;

7 the prevention of hazards to life, human functioning, and human well-being;
8 the promotion of human functioning and development within social groups in accord with human potential, known human limitations and the human desire to be normal (normacy).

These universal self-care requisites embrace the essential physical, psychological, social and spiritual elements of life. Each is important to human functioning. The maintenance of sufficient air, water and food, and provision for elimination, are fundamental to our life process. Problems occurring in these areas could lead to potentially life-threatening conditions. A balance between activity and rest is important in avoiding problems of exhaustion, fatigue or potentially harmful stress. Social interaction is important to the socialisation of individuals into their culture, as well as in providing an opportunity to exchange ideas and opinions. Social interaction also provides the necessary warmth and closeness essential for normal human development. There is a practical importance to social interaction, too, in that social skills may be required in obtaining materials necessary for life, including foods. Solitude is also a prominent consideration, as it provides an opportunity for individuals to reflect and think about their existence and that of others, as well as about the environment surrounding them.

The prevention of hazards to life is essential if an individual is to survive, as well as being a prerequisite to human development. Part of human development necessitates that individuals learn what situations are potentially hazardous, and are able to remove themselves from such environments. Finally, there is a human tendency to be 'normal'. This is derived from genetic and cultural characteristics, as well as known human limitations. *Normacy*, as Orem terms this tendency, involves an individual having a realistic self-concept and being able to cultivate his own development. Additionally, it can refer to an individual being 'accepted' into a peer group or society in general. Taking action to maintain health is considered part of normacy as well as identifying and attending to, where possible, changes in health. This requisite requires an individual to seek and take appropriate action when health, emotional or other problems occur.

These universal self-care requisites are the essential tasks that an individual must be able to manage in order to be self-caring. These eight requisites should not be considered in isolation, however, as they interact. For example, the prevention of hazards should be

7

viewed in the context of all the other requisites – although maintaining a sufficient intake of air, water and food is essential, for instance, awareness of possible toxic and noxious substances must also be considered.

Health-care demands and human ability

Self-care for the average, healthy individual can be viewed in terms of balancing several factors. On the one hand there is the need to be self-caring; universal self-care requisites must be met. On the other hand, the individual must have the ability to satisfy or meet the demands placed upon him. Orem views the universal self-care requisites as self-care demands placed upon an individual: an individual must actively meet these demands through the use of abilities which have been learned and which have an appropriate cultural context. This idea of *balancing* demands and abilities is central to Orem's model, not just at the conceptual level but also in terms of the practical care of patients (Figure 1.1). The use of 'balances' to describe aspects of Orem's model has been adapted from an idea of Aggleton and Chalmers (1986).

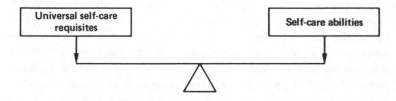

Figure 1.1 *A healthy person: self-care abilities to meet universal self-care requisites*

Developmental self-care requisites

In addition to the universal self-care requisites, essential for all people at every stage of their development, Orem has identified a second kind of requisites found in special circumstances associated with human development (Orem 1991, p.130). These *developmental self-care requisites* have two major classifications.

8

Specific developmental stages

Some developmental requisites relate to bringing about and maintaining conditions that support life processes and promote development – that is, human progress towards higher levels of organisation of human structures and towards maturation. This set of self-care requisites is associated with specific developmental stages, such as being a neonate. At such stages special consideration must be given to aspects of care necessary to the support of life and specifically targeted at promoting development. Specific developmental stages include:

- inter-uterine life and birth;
- neonatal life, whether born to term or prematurely, or of normal or low birth weight;
- infancy;
- the developmental stages of childhood, adolescence and early adulthood;
- the developmental stages of adulthood;
- pregnancy in either childhood or adulthood.

Orem argues that at each of these developmental stages universal self-care requisites must be considered, but there may also be specific health-care demands because of the prevailing developmental level of the individual. An example would be the neonate and temperature regulation: whereas healthy adults are able to manage the control of their own body temperature, for developmental reasons a neonate requires assistance in meeting this need.

✶ Conditions affecting human development

The second set of developmental self-care requisites involves the provision of care associated with the effects of conditions that can adversely affect human development. This developmental self-care requisite has two subtypes.

The first subtype concerns the provision of care to prevent the occurence of deleterious effects of these adverse conditions: examples include the provision of adequate nutrition and rest during pregnancy. Orem is also concerned about the possible hazard to life and development of toxic materials found in the environment.

The second subtype concerns the provision of care to mitigate or overcome existing (or potential) deleterious effects of particular conditions or life events. Examples here include responses to

9

specific life events, such as becoming a parent, or to changes in social and economic conditions. The key consideration is the provision of care to lessen the adverse effects of these conditions on human development. Relevant conditions include:

- educational deprivation;
- problems of social adaptation;
- the loss of relatives, friends or associates;
- the loss of possessions or one's job;
- a sudden change in living conditions;
- a change in status, either social or economic;
- poor health, poor living conditions, or disability;
- terminal illness or expected death;
- environmental hazards.

This consitutes a very wide range of events identified by Orem as being important to the natural process of development of an individual. Being subjected to any one or a combination of these conditions could place increased demands upon the individual's ability to manage his own self-care needs. For example, educational deprivation might inhibit or prevent an individual from developing the necessary skills in seeking information and assistance when this is needed.

Health-deviation self-care requisites

There is one further set of self-care requisites in Orem's model: the *health-deviation self-care requisites* (Orem 1991, p.132). These requisites exist when individuals are ill, become injured, have disabilities, or are under medical care. Under these circumstances, the following additional health-care demands are placed upon an individual:

1 seeking and securing appropriate medical assistance in the event of exposure to specific physical or biological agents or environmental conditions associated with human pathological events and states, or when there is evidence of genetic, physiological, or psychological conditions known to produce, or be associated with, human pathology;

2 being aware of and attending to the effects and results of pathological conditions and states, including effects on development;

3 effectively carrying out medically prescribed diagnostic, therapeutic, and rehabilitative measures directed to preventing specific

types of pathology, to the pathology itself, to the regulation of human integrated functioning, to the correction of deformities or abnormalities, or to compensation for disabilities;

4 being aware of, and attending to or regulating, the discomforting or deleterious effects of medical care measures performed or prescribed by the physician, including effects on development;

5 modifying the self-concept (and self-image) in accepting oneself as being in a particular state of health and in need of specific forms of health care;

6 learning to live with the effects of pathological conditions and states, and the effects of medical diagnostic and treatment measures, in a lifestyle that promotes continued personal development.

The major premise of health-care deviation self-care requisites is that changes in health status require an individual to seek advice and assistance from others competent to offer it when he himself is unable to manage his own self-care needs. It is expected that the person will then comply with any legitimate therapeutic intervention offered to him. Orem recognises that altering one's self-concept may be an important part of becoming unwell, and that it is essential to adapt to changes brought about by illness or injury.

Preventive health care

Orem stresses the importance of preventive health care as an essential component of her model (Orem 1991, p.194). The effective meeting of universal self-care requisites appropriate for an individual is considered to be *primary* prevention. *Secondary* prevention is viewed as the avoidance, by early detection and prompt intervention, of the adverse effects or complications of disease or prolonged disability; while *tertiary* prevention occurs when rehabilitation takes place following disfigurement or disability. These views are in keeping with nursing's increased concerns with health rather than illness.

Overview of self-care requirements

As a broad overview, individuals able to manage their own self-care can:

- support essential physical, psychological and social life processes;
- maintain human structure and function;

- develop their human potential to its fullest;
- prevent injury or disease;
- cure or regulate disease (with appropriate assistance);
- cure or regulate the effects of disease (with appropriate assistance).

These basic tasks will be important later when considering the assessment of the patient.

SELF-CARE DEFICIT

Apart from the natural and everyday need to survive, additional demands on an individual's ability to look after himself can come from many sources. Recent or chronic ill health, or experiencing emotional trauma, may require a person to take further measures to look after himself or seek assistance from others (Orem 1991, p.70). Individuals can have varying abilities to meet the demands placed upon them in performing self-care activities. Healthy people managing their own lives without illness or without the assistance of others are likely to be meeting all their day-to-day self-care needs. People who have existing illness or disease, who have experienced emotional trauma or who have not sufficiently learned or developed self-care skills, may have only a limited ability to meet their self-care needs.

Human beings have a great ability to adapt to changes within themselves and in the environment around them. However, a situation can exist where the total demand placed upon the individual exceeds his ability to meet it. In this situation an individual may need help to meet self-care needs; assistance can come from many sources, including relatives, friends and nursing interventions.

The idea of balance, used in Figure 1.1 to portray the relationship between health-care demands and self-care abilities, can be used again to depict the idea of *self-care deficit*. There are three scenarios which demonstrate how an individual's ability to manage self-care can be influenced by increased demands being placed upon him.

Consider first a healthy individual, able to manage all self-care demands, who catches a cold. In this situation, superimposed upon this person's usual system of looking after himself there is now an additional health need – a health-deviation self-care requisite. The cold-related effects may influence the ability to self-care; there may be tiredness, lack of motivation, and a need for solitude. There is also the requirement to use learned knowledge and skills to seek appropriate advice and assistance and to comply with this informa-

12

tion. Suitable action might be to do nothing, or perhaps to use home remedies or visit one's general practitioner. Whatever course is decided upon, the result must be a conscious and deliberate action. However, a relatively minor irritation over a cold is unlikely to require assistance. The ability of the healthy individual to seek information, make health judgements and take appropriate action can indicate that an individual is managing his own care satisfactorily (Figure 1.2).

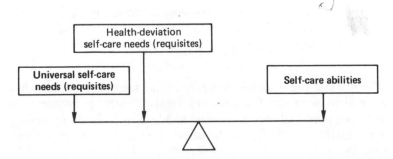

Figure 1.2 *An individual experiencing a change in health status but still able to meet universal and health-deviation self-care requisites*

Now consider an otherwise healthy individual who has sustained a fractured limb. In this situation a person would need to seek competent assistance, including nursing assistance, to meet universal self-care requisites (Figure 1.3): his self-care abilities would be inadequate. Consider the universal self-care requisites that could be influenced due to a fractured leg. There might be difficulty in obtaining sufficient nutrients; elimination could be a problem, as could achieving suitable rest, because of pain. Being hospitalised could interfere with the normal social processes the person would otherwise engage in, such as meeting friends or being involved in various activities. These issues might be compounded by the developmental level of the patient. A young child might experience separation anxiety due to being away from his parents, while an elderly person might need special attention to deal with the possibility of being disorientated in an unfamiliar environment. Whatever the situation, health-deviation self-care requisites must be attended to, in particular following medical and nursing advice as well as dealing with changes in body-image or self-concept and learning to manage effectively, or to adapt to, the current situation.

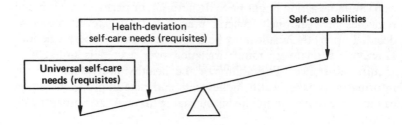

Figure 1.3 *An individual experiencing a change in health status, unable to meet universal and health-deviation self-care requisites and so needing nursing intervention*

Continuing the situation above, the third scenario is found when the patient with the fractured leg receives nursing assistance in managing universal, developmental and health-deviation requisites. Immediately after the injury the person is unlikely to be self-caring. However, part of the process of becoming self-caring is showing the ability to adapt and to change current life practices to ones more suited to new situations – in this case that of becoming a patient (Figure 1.4).

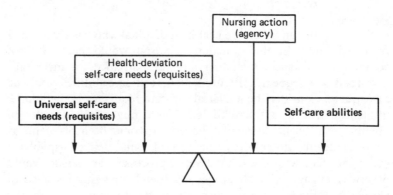

Figure 1.4 *An individual able to meet universal and health-deviation self-care requisites with nursing assistance*

While the use of balances to 'weigh out' the relationship between the demands on a patient to be self-caring and his actual ability to meet these (with or without assistance) is a helpful model, care should be taken in interpreting such comparisons. Orem herself does not specifically use this approach to demonstrate relationships; and aspects of the model such as the angle of slope of the differences between demands and abilities have no meaning – this is simply a visual model.

In summary, self-care deficits are a way of describing the relationship between the abilities of individuals to act and the demands on them for self-care, or for care of children or adults who are their dependents (Orem 1991, p.73). The 'deficit' must be seen as the relationship between an individual's abilities and the demands placed upon him: it is not itself a disorder, although the individual may also have physical and psychological problems.

Therapeutic self-care demand

The *therapeutic self-care demand* is the set of self-care actions needed in order to meet known self-care requisites (Orem 1991, p.123). Therapeutic self-care demand can be viewed as a 'summary statement' of the relationship between the self-care requisites known to exist for a patient (or those that may occur in the future) and what can or should be done to meet them. A statement of an individual's therapeutic self-care demand is therefore a description of the individual, in terms of his development, structure and function.

Self-care agency

Orem uses the word 'agent' to refer to the person who actually provides care or takes some specific action (Orem 1991, p.154). When individuals provide their own care, they are considered to be *self-care agents*. The ability of individuals to participate in their own self-care is called their *self-care agency*.

For the average healthy person engaged in carrying out his own self-care activities, self-care agency is present in a developed or developing form. Individuals who know how to manage their own health needs are considered to have developed a self-care agency able to meet self-care needs. In other situations self-care agency is still developing, as with children who are becoming toilet-trained – there are increasing development of sphincter control and increasing understanding of the elimination process; and this learning takes place within culturally defined limits. Thirdly, individuals may have a developed self-care agency that is nevertheless not functioning. For example, a person might realise that he is in need of aid, be capable of seeking assistance but choose *not* to find help, perhaps because of fear or anxiety.

Dependent-care agency

Orem recognises that situations do occur when people care for each other without directly involving nursing care. This concept is called *dependent-care agency*. In essence, this is the ability of some mature people to recognize that others (such as children, adolescents or adults with health-related limitations) have self-care requisites that they themselves cannot meet, and to meet some or all of these on their behalf (Orem 1991, p.175). In the situation of adults looking after children and young people, the emphasis is on the meeting or modifying of universal, developmental or health-deviation self-care requisites, and on developing caring or parenting activities.

Adults may become involved in a wide range of dependent-care activities, providing either complete or partial care. Consider a newborn baby unable as yet to meet such needs as the ability to obtain food, or a patient in a coma unable to manage many basic life functions. In these situations a parent or nurse will adopt the caring role and help to meet universal, developmental and health-deviation self-care requisites. Orem describes an individual who provides care to others to meet their self-care needs as the *dependent-care agent*; in the situation of the nurse providing care, it is nursing agency that is being used.

CARING FOR ONESELF

The act of caring for oneself requires the initiation of a complex series of behaviours, behaviours necessitating a personal and deliberate approach to self-care. The process of self-caring starts with being aware of one's health condition. This awareness itself requires rational thought in drawing upon personal experience, cultural norms and learned behaviours in order to make a decision about one's health status. There must also be a conscious desire to want to meet one's own self-care needs; this is an important assumption underlying Orem's model. When a decision has been reached to adopt certain self-care behaviours in response to a specific need, a definite plan or procedure for action must be devised to meet this perceived need. Once decided upon, there must be a willingness and commitment to continue with the plan.

The ability to be self-caring relies upon the individual having learned much about himself, the nature of health, and cultural expectations. In order to be self-caring an individual must possess the following:

1 Ability to maintain attention and exercise requisite vigilance with respect to self as self-care agent and internal and external conditions and factors significant for self-care.
2 Controlled use of available physical energy that is sufficient for the initiation and continuation of self-care operations.
3 Ability to control the position of the body and its parts in the execution of the movements required for the initiation and completion of self-care operations.
4 Ability to reason within a self-care frame of reference.
5 Motivation (i.e., goal orientations for self-care that are in accord with its characteristics and its meaning for life, health, and well-being).
6 Ability to make decision about care of self and to operationalize these decisions.
7 Ability to acquire technical knowledge about self-care from authoritative sources, to retain it, and to operationalize it.
8 A repertoire of cognitive, perceptual, manipulative, communication, and interpersonal skills adapted to the performance of self-care operations.
9 Ability to order discrete self-care actions or action systems into relationships with prior and subsequent actions toward the final achievement of regulatory goals of self-care.
10 Ability to consistently perform self-care operations, integrating them with relevant aspects of personal, family, and community living.

(Orem 1991, p.155)

Self-care limitations

An individual with these abilities is likely to be able to meet his own self-care needs. However, there can be barriers or limitations to self-care. The person may lack knowledge about himself and perhaps have no desire to find out. There may be difficulties in making health judgements; just when is it time to seek the advice and assistance of others? There may be difficulties in learning about the self or about the actions required in order to be self-caring. There may be problems in participating in the planning and delivery of care, because of physical, psychological or emotional disabilities (Orem 1991, p. 169).

What is a patient?

Orem's work is important because it attempts to establish the boundaries of nursing action – when is nursing required, and (once initiated) when can nursing action cease? Generally, however, a patient is an individual who requires nursing assistance to meet specific self-care demands, and this assistance can redress or overcome a limited ability (Orem 1991, p.30). Orem's definition of 'patient', from the nursing perspective, requires three conditions to be satisfied:

1 There must be some self-care demand (universal, developmental or health-deviation) to be met for another person. This suggests that if a person can manage his own self-care, nursing assistance will not be required. This is not always as straightforward as it may seem, however: cultural and social differences may lead to differences of opinion regarding whether assistance is actually required, and before care can be offered an individual must have some health knowledge and the ability to make the decision to seek aid.
2 Some self-care ability must be either present or potential (available for development in the future). There must be some desire on the part of an individual to want to become self-caring, or an expectation that after suitable medical and nursing interventions, the individual will be able to adopt some self-caring behaviours. For example, the patient with a spinal injury may have limited self-care abilities now, but following suitable interventions may be expected to take an increasing role in self-care.
3 A deficit relationship must exist between a person's self-care demands and his ability to meet those demands – that is, an individual is not currently able to meet his self-care requisites by himself, or there is a likelihood of his not being able to do so in the future. Thus, a patient with a degenerative joint condition may be able to manage day-to-day care now, but as the condition develops nursing assistance may be needed.

The nature of nursing action

Nurses can perform many functions to assist patients. Orem has classified these actions into five categories (Orem 1991, p.286), which may be expressed thus:

1 to act or do for others;
2 to guide or direct others;
3 to support, either physically or psychologically;
4 to provide an appropriate environment for care to be delivered and personal abilities to be developed;
5 to teach.

Perhaps the most obvious function of nurses is in acting on behalf of another who is unable to perform a specific health-care task. However, while this may cover the traditional physical caring tasks which nurses perform there are many other responsibilities placed upon the nurse. Guiding and directing the patient is a role that requires her to provide information or advice relevant to the patient to help meet his self-care needs. The giving of physiological and psychological support is another important nursing role. Physical support can be viewed as a partnership – a cooperative team of patient, nurse and others meeting agreed health-care needs – while Orem views psychological support as the provision of an 'understanding presence', a person able to listen and to offer a variety of methods to help the patient. The environment is very important in the care of the patient, and the nurse is charged with providing an environment which is conducive to meeting the patient's health-care needs, and which will assist the patient in developing new abilities and prevent new limitations from occurring. Finally, the nurse must be a teacher. This role requires that nurses have knowledge and skills themselves and are able to communicate these to others. Specifically, a nurse must be able to describe and explain to the patient his self-care demands, the methods and courses of action or treatment needed to meet his self-care needs, ways of managing his self-care, and methods of compensating for limitations in his ability to self-care. These actions are not mutually exclusive; there may be many instances where several different types of nursing action are being initiated simultaneously to meet a specific health goal. The giving of physical care, for example, may be accompanied by discussion with the patient about his care, and education to prevent future difficulties.

THE NURSING PROCESS

Orem has stressed throughout her model that nursing is action, and, as with other nursing models, ideas must be translated into a form that can be utilised in practice (Orem 1991, p.269). Translation is achieved using the nursing process, a method traditionally consisting of four stages: assessment, planning, intervention, and evaluation. Orem advocates the use of a nursing process, but in a way more consistent with her theory. Specifically, she views the nursing process as one requiring nurses to participate in *interpersonal and social operations* and *technologic-professional operations.*

Interpersonal and social operations

Interpersonal and social processes involve the nurse developing an appropriate social and interpersonal style when working with patients and their families. In particular, nurses should:

- begin and maintain an effective relationship with the patient, his family and others;
- agree with the patient and others to answer health-related questions;
- continually collaborate and review information with the patient and others.

The processes must be maintained or modified, where appropriate, throughout nursing relationships with patients.

Technologic-professional operations

Technologic-professional operations are identified as *diagnostic, prescriptive, treatment or regulatory,* and *case-management operations.* While there is an inherent sequence to these operations, in that logically diagnostic (assessment) actions must occur prior to prescriptive (planning) actions, it is possible for care to be initiated and evaluated (treatment or regulatory operations) before all the required assessment information has been obtained. Case-management operations, however (the care-audit aspects of the nursing process), will continue throughout nursing interaction with patients. Orem views the technologic-professional operations as 'milestones' in the nursing process but recognises that the performance of these operations will be dependent on the patient, his family, the nurse, and possibly other factors. The technologic-professional operations are particular to Orem's model, and worth looking at in detail.

Nursing diagnosis

This operation may have a medically-orientated connotation, but for Orem (1991, p.270) nursing diagnosis involves the investigation and accumulation of facts about a patient's self-care ability and his self-care demands, and the nature of the relationship between the two. Essentially, the nursing diagnosis determines whether the patient is in need of nursing assistance, and can be equated with the assessment stage of the more familiar 'nursing process' format (Figure 1.5).

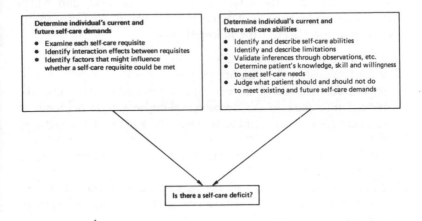

Figure 1.5 *Nursing diagnosis (assessment)*

More specifically, the nursing diagnosis is likely to involve addressing two issues:

Current and future self-care demand

What is the patient's current self-care demand, and what is it likely to be in the future? The calculation of a person's self-care demand follows a logical process of examining the patient's condition in the light of the universal, developmental and health-deviation self-care requisites. This process can be summarised in the following way:

1 examine each universal, developmental or health-deviation self-care requisite to determine whether any current problems exist and whether there is the potential for future problems;
2 identify possible interaction effects between universal, developmental and health-deviation self-care requisites;
3 identify factors that might influence whether a self-care requisite could be met.

21

Current and future self-care ability

Can the patient meet these self-care demands? It is necessary to determine whether the patient can manage his own self-care, not just in terms of present practice but also for the future. An assessment must be made of the repertoire of knowledge and skills that he has with which to meet daily self-care demands. To achieve this, one must identify which health practices the patient is able to perform without assistance, which will need to be developed, and which should cease. This process of determining a patient's self-care ability can be put into effect in the following ways:

1 identify and describe the patient's range of self-care practices;
2 identify and describe limitations;
3 make inferences about the general abilities and limitations of the patient to engage in the decision-making and actions phases of self-care (that is, determine whether the patient has a self-care deficit);
4 validate inferences through observation, measurement, and the like;
5 determine the adequacy of the patient's knowledge, skills and willingness to meet each self-care requisite using named methods and measures of care;
6 judge what the patient is able to do, not able to do, and should do to meet existing self-care demands presently and in the future;
7 when a self-care deficit exists, identify what the patient should and should not do in the immediate meeting of self-care demands;
8 in the event of an existing or potential self-care deficit, determine the patient's future capabilities to develop the necessary health-care skills.

Prescriptive operations

Prescriptive operations are the practical judgements that must be taken by nurse and patient following the collection of data, and can be equated with the 'planning' phase of the traditional nursing process. These operations address the issues of what can be done for the individual given his present circumstances and knowledge. It also considers what could happen in the future. Orem stresses that prescriptive operations must be considered in the light of the *totality* of the individual and not in relation to single pieces of information. Prescriptive operations specify the following aspects of care (see Orem 1991, p.271):

1 the means to be used to meet particular self-care requisites, and the courses of actions, or care measures, to be performed to meet these requisites;
2 the totality of care measures to be performed to meet all components of the therapeutic self-care demand, including a good organization of these care measures;
3 the roles of the nurse(s), the patient and the dependent-care agent(s) in meeting the therapeutic self-care demand;
4 the roles of the nurse(s), the patient and the dependent-care agent(s) in regulating the exercise or development of self-care agency.

The prescriptive operation involves the bringing together of both the interpersonal and social processes of nursing with technologic-professional roles. For example, interpersonal processes may involve collaborating with patients or relatives over the giving of information, or reaching agreements on the timing of giving care; while technologic-professional operations include specifying the methods to meet a particular self-care requisite. These series of nursing operations are seen as occurring concurrently. In other words, while more 'technical' aspects of care are being planned and carried out there is a requirement on nursing to develop and maintain good interpersonal and social contact with the patient and his family.

Orem stresses the importance of involving family members and significant others in the overall prescription process. It is recognised that some people will want to take a full and active part in their own self-care or the dependent-care of others, while some relatives may be psychologically unprepared to care for others. Thus Orem suggests that nurses should attempt to identify the personality characteristics of patients and relatives that may affect the nursing situation – for example, passivity or grief – and explore concerns that may interfere with collaboration with nursing staff. To do this nurses need to make observations and use subjective information elicited during their assessments.

Regulatory or treatment operations

Regulatory or treatment operations are the practical activities which are undertaken to carry out what has been prescribed earlier. Particularly important is the development of an appropriate system (an orderly arrangement) for the delivery of care. Regulatory and treatment operations can be equated to the 'intervention' and 'evaluation' components of the traditional nursing process.

Designs for regulatory operations: the nursing system

The design of a *nursing system* (Orem 1991, p.276): includes the following tasks:

1 Create a system of relationships to meet self-care requirements now and in the future.
2 Specify the timing and amount of nurse–patient contact, and the reasons for it.
3 Identify the contributions of both the nurse and the patient in meeting self-care demands, ensuring that:
   (a) there is a routine of self-care tasks, and a time sequence for completing them;
   (b) there is regulation of the amount that patients engage in their own self-care;
   (c) patients develop an interest in their own care and the desire to become self-caring;
   (d) patients develop, refine or master existing self-care skills;
   (e) patients develop new skills and abilities in meeting self-care needs, without developing new limitations.

Nursing is the action performed by nurses, for the benefit of others, to meet specific health goals. Once the nurse has established that a nursing situation exists, the way in which she organises her endeavours and approaches to the care of a patient is extremely important. The manner and context in which a nurse and a patient interact is called a *nursing system* (Orem 1991, p.285). The basic elements constituting a nursing system are:

1 the nurse(s);
2 the patient or a group of people;
3 the events occurring between them, including interaction with relatives and friends.

All nursing systems have several things in common, in particular these:

- the reasons for having a nursing relationship must be clearly established;
- the general and specific roles of the nurse, patient and significant others must be determined;
- the scope of nursing responsibility must be determined;
- the specific action to be adopted to meet specific health-care needs must be stated;
- action required to regulate self-care ability in meeting self-care demands in the future must be estimated.

24

Orem considers there to be three types of nursing systems: *wholly compensatory, partly compensatory*, and *supportive-educative* (Figure 1.6).

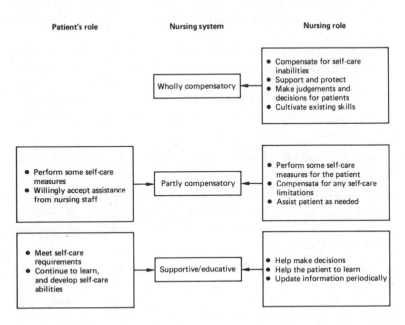

Figure 1.6 *Nursing systems*

Wholly compensatory   The type of nursing system required when the nurse performs a major compensatory role for the patient (Orem 1991, p.289): often the patient is unable to meet his own universal self-care requisites and the nurse must manage these until such time as the patient can resume his own care (if possible) or until he has learned to adapt to any disability. This nursing system is required in each of the following situations:

1 The patient appears unable to engage in any form of deliberate self-care action, as for example when in a coma. Generally, any person who is unable to control his movements, or appears to be unresponsive to a wide variety of stimuli (auditory, visual, tactile, etc.), or is unable to communicate with others will require a wholly compensatory system.
2 The patient is aware of the need to engage in self-care activities, is able to make health judgements and take decisions and has the skills to do so, but cannot or should not make actions requiring

25

ambulation or manipulative movements. Other characteristics may include being aware of himself and his environment and being able to communicate with others, although this ability may be greatly restricted. An example of this is a person on strict bed rest following a cerebrovascular accident, and subject to expressive aphasia.

3 The patient is unable to attend to his own health-care needs, make reasoned judgements or take decisions, but can perform manipulative and ambulatory movements. This would be true for an individual who had just started to regain consciousness following surgery, or an individual with impaired judgement following a head injury.

Generally, the nurse's role in wholly compensatory nursing systems is:

- to compensate for self-care inabilities a patient may have;
- to support and protect the patient while providing an environment suitable for cultivating existing self-care skills and fostering the development of new ones.

Nurses must not only be the providers of care but must also make the necessary judgements and take decisions on behalf of the patient. This responsibility extends to the universal, developmental and health-care deviation self-care requisites.

Partly compensatory This type of nursing system does not require the same breadth and intensity of nursing intervention as the wholly compensatory nursing system (Orem 1991, p.291). The nurse must still act in a compensatory role, but the patient is much more involved in his own care in terms of decision-making and action. Such a nursing system would be appropriate in the following situations:

1 The patient is limited in mobility or manipulative skills, either actually or by medical requirement.
2 The patient has a knowledge or skills deficit, or both, preventing him from meeting all of his self-care needs. An example of this is a person recently developing diabetes mellitus and needing to learn the technical aspects of insulin administration and the lifestyle changes associated with this condition.
3 The patient is not psychologically ready to perform, or to learn to perform, self-care behaviours. This situation is exemplified by a

person who has recently had a limb amputated; it may take some time before he can begin to adapt to his new situation.

The nurse's role in the partly compensatory nursing system may require the use of all five helping methods (page 19) and is likely to include:

- performing some self-care measures for the patient;
- compensating for any self-care limitations a patient may have;
- assisting the patient as required.

This nursing system also places some responsibilities on the patient, including:

- performing some self-care measures (patients are expected to become involved in the management of their own care when they are able to);
- accepting care and assistance from nursing staff where appropriate.

Supportive/educative   This nursing system would be suitable for the patient who is able to perform the actions necessary for self-care, and can learn to adapt to new situations, but currently needs nursing assistance; sometimes this may simply involve giving reassurance (Orem 1991, p.291). Generally, the nurse's role will be limited to helping to make decisions and communicating knowledge and skills. This system may require the nurse to teach the patient, or she may have to manipulate the environment to assist learning, perhaps by reducing unnecessary distractions. A consultative role may exist for the nurse if only periodic information or updating is required. The nurse's role in the supportive/educative nursing system is primarily one of regulating the delivery and development of self-care abilites, while the patient himself accomplishes self-care.

These nursing systems should not be viewed as just another way of classifying patients, once assigned never to be changed. Nursing systems need to be dynamic, as is illustrated in care planning. A patient may initially require a wholly compensatory nursing system to meet universal self-care requisites; as his condition changes so does the nursing system needed. A partly compensatory system would be suitable for a patient who is becoming increasingly involved in his own care, and ultimately a supportive/educative system may be warranted. Nursing systems can also overlap; a partly compensatory *and* supportive/educative nursing system is appropriate when the patient must acquire both knowledge and skills.

Nursing action

Following the decision to adopt a particular system, or part of a system, the nurse is in a position to decide how best to achieve patient care goals. The general methods that can be used, described earlier, include performing tasks for the patient, helping to guide and direct others, offering physical or psychological support, providing a suitable environment for the patient to continue to develop, and patient education.

Planning for regulatory operations

Planning is seen by Orem as adding practical and resource implications to the nursing system. In particular, planning adds the following dimensions.

Time A timeframe is important when planning care and stating patient goals. The use of a realistic timeframe can help to determine whether an intervention has been successful or not.

Place The venue for the delivery of care depends upon the nature of the patient's self-care demand, his ability to meet this demand, and his self-care limitations. It may be appropriate, for example, to teach an individual how to self-administer insulin in his own home rather than having to go to an artificial setting such as the hospital or clinic.

Environmental conditions This may be important for the provision of rest and the avoidance of undue stress. A patient recently experiencing an intra-cranial bleed may need to have the environment strictly controlled to provide quietness, subdued lighting, and restricted contact with others.

Equipment and supplies Ensuring the appropriate equipment and supplies necessary for a nursing intervention is extremely important.

Decisions will have to be made about the availibility of equipment and cost-effectiveness.

The number and qualification of staff needed to conduct, evaluate and modify the care plan Some aspects of care, by their very nature, will determine the manpower requirements needed to achieve health goals. An ill neonate will demand staff who are technologically skilled, while the community psychiatric nurse's care will be focused on interpersonal skills.

Regulatory care

Nurses help patients to meet their self-care needs, and regulate the exercise or development of abilities to engage in self-care. This operation is ultimately the 'doing and thinking' aspect of nursing (Orem 1991, p.280). In this respect Orem is prescriptive, giving clear guidance concerning what nurses should be doing, but also what should be charted by nurses in their day-to-day reporting about patients. These activities include the following:

1 Perform and regulate the self-care tasks of patients or assist patients with their performance of self-care tasks.
2 Coordinate the performance of self-care tasks.
3 Help patients, their families, and others establish an appropriate environment for daily living that supports the accomplishment of self-care, but also satisfies the patient's interest, talents, and goals.
4 Guide, support or direct patients in their exercise, or withholding of their self-care agency.
5 Stimulate patients' interest in self-care by raising questions and promoting discussions of care problems and issues when conditions permit.
6 Support and guide patients in learning activities and provide cues for learning as well as instructional sessions.
7 Support and guide patients as they experience illness or disability and the effects of medical care measures. Continue this support as the patient experiences the need to engage in new activities of self-care, or needs to change their ways of meeting current self-care needs.   (Orem 1991, p.280)

The above points constitute an inventory of the direct nursing care that will be offered to patients. This inventory, however, goes beyond just the physical acts of caring to include all the supportive and educational aspects of care.

Regulatory care-evaluation component

Orem adds three further operations to the above list of nursing actions, because of the need to decide whether nursing care should be continued in the current way or whether changes are needed. These last three nursing actions require the nurse to make judgements about the existing care plan and the patient's progress in meeting outcomes or goals. Determining progress and evaluating the effect of nursing care given is essential, and Orem offers some specific guidance to nurses, by indicating what should be noted:

8 Monitor patients and assist patients to monitor themselves to determine if self-care measures are performed, and to determine the effects of self-care behaviours.

9 Make judgements about the sufficiency and efficiency of patient self-care, the patient's ability to develop their own self-care skill repertoire, and nursing assistance.

10 Make judgements about the patient's perceptions of the results obtained through nursing intervention, and make or recommend adjustments in the nursing care system through changes in nurse and patient roles.

Manifest here is the importance of obtaining feedback from patients about *their* perceptions of how care is progressing, rather than just from nursing or other health staff, and the need to consider making changes in the care plan. This aspect of Orem's view of the care-planning directs nurses to assess the effectiveness of their plan and make changes – a feedback mechanism.

Case-management (control) operations

Case-management operations are concerned with the evaluation, control, directing and checking of each of the diagnostic, prescriptive, treatment and regulatory operations specific for the individual. Case management is particularly important in that it integrates all aspects of nursing care, ensuring that there is a dynamic process and response to changes within the patient. Additionally, it ensures that resources are used wisely and that any psychological or physical stresses that a person might encounter while receiving or seeking care are minimised. Essentially, the control aspects of the nursing process involve not just the evaluation of care but also an audit of resource utilisation.

Specifically, control operations include observation and appraisal, to determine:

1 if regulatory or treatment operations are performed periodically or continuously according to the design for the system of nursing under production for a patient;

2 if the operations performed are in accord with the conditions of the patient or the patient's environment for the regulation of which they have been prescribed, or if the prescription is no longer valid; and

3 if regulation of the patient's functioning is being achieved through performance of care measures to meet the patient's therapeutic self-care demand, if the exercise of patient's self-care agency is properly regulated, if developmental change is in process and is adequate, or if the patient is adjusting to declining powers to engage in self-care.

(Orem 1991, p.282)

An overview of the nursing process using Orem's model is presented in Figure 1.7.

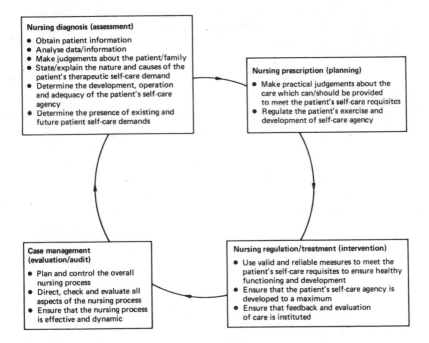

Figure 1.7   *Overview of the nursing process using Orem's model of nursing*

Summary

Orem emphasises that the first part of any nursing process must be to determine whether nursing assistance is required, and that this judgement should be validated by using information from as many sources as possible. This validation is likely to come from a negotiated understanding between professional groups, the individual and his family. Once it has been determined that nursing assistance and intervention is appropriate, nurses must design a system of nursing care that will achieve the health goals determined for that particular patient. Once designed there is a phase of implementation which focuses on helping to compensate for health-care limitations, encouraging existing abilities and preventing new limitations.

This chapter has examined some of the key components of Orem's model of nursing. Reference has been made to the practical application of the model to nursing situations. Part II of this book offers a series of care studies which utilise the model as a foundation. Following each study are questions, exercises or other activities to supplement the readings.

PART II

Applying the model

CHAPTER TWO

Planning care

THEORY INTO PRACTICE

This section presents a series of nursing care plans based upon Orem's model of nursing. Preparing care plans is an essential aspect of current nursing practice, and using a nursing model can pose special challenges. While Orem has given direction regarding the way in which nursing and patient care can develop, she has left it to the individual nurse to determine how to adopt and work with the model. This suggests that there is no single 'correct' method of setting out a plan based upon Orem's model. Instead, the nurse must take Orem's ideas and use them in whatever way is appropriate to develop a plan of care that will meet each patient's needs.

This is not to suggest that there is no logic in planning care; Orem's ideas do require a considerable amount of work in gathering appropriate assessment data and in crafting a plan. The result of this is that a variety of formats and organisational layouts can be used to plan care. This in itself can be ambiguous: it would be very much easier if there were an agreed format used by everybody who used Orem's model, but such a format simply does not exist.

The care plans that follow are not intended to be 'perfect'; the dynamic nature of nursing requires a plan to be reviewed, and possibly changed, regularly. Rather they represent a variety of ways in which Orem's ideas can be harnessed to plan, organise, deliver and evaluate care. By offering a variety of approaches, different aspects of Orem's model can be introduced, and key aspects of her model illustrated. Additionally, this demonstration of the potential for variety and flexibility in preparing a care plan may help to dispel the notion that there are practical constraints requiring one model format to be adopted. Indeed, there can be many creative uses of

Orem's ideas, all leading to workable care plans. It is hoped that the range of patient scenarios used in this part of the book will allow you to identify with some common situations likely to be experienced either while training or as a qualified nurse.

The Orem model readily follows the nursing process of assessment, planning, intervention and evaluation. The theoretical details of Orem's understanding of each of these processes, presented in Chapter 1, need to be linked to their practical application. This is essential if Orem is to make any meaningful contribution to nursing practice and patient care. One approach to this problem is to identify the key clinical behaviours which constitute nursing practice based on Orem; specifically, the key questions or behaviours which should be considered by nurses who are using Orem's model to plan care. Because of their different circumstances, not every patient will need all of the following questions addressed. The following lists, which may provide useful guidance in planning actual care, have been adapted from the work of Dorothy Reilly and Marilyn Oermann (1985).

GUIDANCE IN PLANNING

Background information

1 Evaluate the biological, social, psychological, and cultural influences on the patient's ability to care for himself.
2 Identify the impact of the patient's condition on his own natural development.
3 Identify and analyse the impact of the patient's condition on family members and on their interaction.
4 Identify the patient's and his family's needs for information, and their ability to learn.
5 Identify and analyse the patient's potential to be self-caring.

Assessment

1 Perform a thorough and systematic assessment of the patient.
2 Evaluate the impact of the patient's condition on his lifestyle.
3 Identify the current coping strategies adopted by the patient.
4 Appraise the impact of biopsychosocial and cultural factors on the patient's response to his condition.
5 Identify the developmental level of the patient and his family.

6 Identify the support systems available to the patient.
7 From the patient assessment, calculate the therapeutic self-care demand of the patient.
8 Identify the nature of any self-care deficits in relation to the patient's condition, and the reasons why they exist.
9 Identify and analyse the learning needs of the patient and his family.
10 Develop nursing care objectives based upon the identified self-care deficits.

Planning

1 Develop patient care goals that are consistent with the patient's identified needs.
2 Plan the nursing management of care, aimed at overcoming the patient's self-care deficits and those problems that the patient's family may be encountering.
3 Support the patient's own decision-making in relation to his care.
4 Identify and select appropriate methods to manage the patient's self-care deficits.
5 Provide the appropriate resources required for the care of the patient, including equipment and personnel.

Implementation

1 Implement nursing interventions consistent with a scientific rationale, research and a mutually established plan of care.
2 Initiate referrals to health-care providers and/or agencies essential in assisting the patient to meet his optimum self-care agency.
3 Encourage the patient in the use of his own potential and resources in addressing self-care limitations.
4 Protect the patient's self-care abilities as a means of preventing new self-care limitations.
5 Document pertinent nursing observations and interventions.

Evaluation

1 Develop criteria for evaluating the effectiveness of the plan in moving towards a decrease in self-care deficit and an increase in self-care agency.

2 Use these criteria in evaluating the patient and family outcomes of care in terms of stated goals.
3 Use professional nursing standards as a framework for evaluating the process of the delivery of nursing care.
4 Modify the plan of care as appropriate to the evaluation results.

CHAPTER THREE

Care study: recovery from a stroke

JOHN

John is a 63-year-old man who has been in good health for most of his life, not even having been hospitalised as a child. While not seeking medical assistance regularly, he is interested in health-related issues, in particular diet. He would prefer to pay a little extra for fresh fruit and vegetables and leaner cuts of meat. He has been an active individual, playing cricket as a member of the local team; living on the south coast has provided plenty of opportunities to walk and to feel the freshness of the sea breeze, which he loves.

He has never married, but maintains a close network of friends from his work and from the cricket team, even out of season. Like John, many of his friends are academics. He enjoys sitting with them and debating current affairs, as well as history, his specialist interest. He likes to drink with them but doesn't smoke. During work time he is fairly sedentary but looks forward to weekends, when he can explore the countryside.

John is fortunate in that he has no financial worries. He inherited his house from his parents when they died, and he is careful with his money. He employs a housekeeper, who cleans three times a week and does some of the shopping for him.

Catastrophe

John is found on the floor of his house about midday on a Monday. His housekeeper, who finds him, calls the ambulance service which takes him to the local District General Hospital. Upon admission he is found to be sleepy but easily rousable by auditory stimulation. He is unable to speak intelligibly but appears to understand what is being said to him. It is obvious from examination that he is unable to move the limbs on the right side of his body; these limbs have increased muscle tone. He can move the left side of his body, but has difficulty in performing fine movements. He is unable to stand. John also has a weakness of the lower right part of his face; his lip droops to the right and he is dribbling saliva.

There are no immediate respiratory difficulties and he can cough and deep-breathe spontaneously; his gag reflex appears intact. His blood pressure is moderately elevated (150/95) and his pulse rate is 80. No cardiac arrhythmias are noted while he is having an electrocardiograph. He has been incontinent of urine.

It appears from the history and examination that a vessel or vessels carrying blood in the left side of John's brain has become occluded, resulting in motor weakness affecting his right side including part of his face. The speech centre of the brain – usually in the left cerebral hemisphere of a right-handed person – has also been involved in the lesion: the result appears to be an expressive, but not receptive, aphasia. Some visual disturbance (hemianopia) has occurred, but his hearing has not been affected.

Following this initial accident and the emergency-room examination, John is transported to an acute medical ward. He remains there for two weeks.

ASSESSMENT

Universal self-care requisites

The maintenance of a sufficient intake of air

John is able to breathe without difficulty and to cough and breathe deeply when asked. However, because of difficulties he has in controlling his saliva, there is concern about the risk of choking or of aspirating saliva. Additionally, because of his relatively immobile state, there is the potential for respiratory tract infections.

The maintenance of a sufficient intake of water

John has a right-sided facial weakness and has difficulty controlling his saliva, which dribbles from the side of his mouth. He also appears to have difficulty in swallowing. Due to mobility problems, he is unable to obtain fluids by himself and needs physical assistance in drinking, and observation to ensure that he does not choke. Without prompting, he forgets to have a drink and there is the possibility of his becoming dehydrated.

The maintenance of a sufficient intake of food

There is concern for John because of his apparent dysphagia. He needs assistance to obtain food and to eat. Provided food is puréed and assistance given, he is able to consume foods although he requires close observation at all times. John needs to have a balanced diet presented to him.

The provision of care associated with elimination processes and excrements

John is incontinent of urine most of the time and is unable to void at will. He is also unable to manage his bowel functions. He does not know when he has been incontinent, and part of his sacral area is becoming irritated and sore. With prolonged periods of immobility, urinary tract infections could occur.

The maintenance of a balance between activity and rest

John is quite agitated at times; his mood changes from anger to tearfulness. He is often unable to sleep or to get comfortable. When he does sleep it is only for short periods, and as a result he is becoming increasingly fatigued.

The maintenance of a balance between solitude and social integration

John has difficulties with speech. Being aphasic, the words he utters often do not make sense: this causes him great frustration and anger. He can clearly understand what is being said to him, and indicates to staff when he wants to be left alone by gesturing with his left hand. Sometimes he refuses to see his friends, which is distressing for them.

The prevention of hazards to life, human functioning and human well-being

There are general concerns with John's control of his airway, and he is unstable on his feet. When he attempts to walk, with assistance, his right leg shows some movement but it is uncoordinated and drags behind him. There is the obvious risk of falling. He is also disorientated, particularly as regards the hospital environment, the day, the date and the time. His vital signs were initially found to be elevated, but they are not now abnormal for a man of his age and physical condition.

Normacy

While not being able to express these concerns directly, John is likely to be having some difficulties with his self-esteem and body image. He is frightened, partly because of a new dependency on others but also because of the possible loss of affection from his friends. He needs to develop trust in others, particularly in performing tasks which he has managed himself for most of his life. He is anxious and demoralised by the prospect of staying in hospital for a long time – he wants to go home. There is also a feeling of loss, not just of physiological functioning (of his bladder and bowel), but also of social and economic status. It is speculated that he probably doesn't want to be a burden on anyone else, and this may give rise to feelings of guilt.

Developmental self-care requisites

The process of human development occurs throughout life, and John has undergone changes which have resulted in alterations to the natural process of his development. At the moment, the changes to his social and economic status mean that he can no longer meet his friends in the same way, or participate in the activities he enjoys. This prevents him from cultivating new friendships in the way he has been used to and from participating in activities he enjoys. Furthermore, he will not be able to return to his job in the foreseeable future. John, though he likes his work, has in some ways looked forward to retirement when he would have time for activities that he has not been able to pursue because of his employment commitments. It is not immediately obvious now whether he will indeed be able to do the things he has planned for; nor, if he is unable to, what his reaction to this situation will be.

Health-deviation self-care requisites

John is unable to meet many of the additional demands placed upon him as a result of his illness. In particular:

1 It is difficult to determine the extent of his understanding of his illness.
2 He has difficulty in complying with medical and other health advice. During times of anger or frustration he resents staff trying to help him, particularly at mealtimes and when he has been incontinent. An important intervention is to encourage frequent exercises to increase the mobility of his right side. These sessions are particularly stressful for him. With some right-sided loss of sensation and coordination, movement and managing the tasks of everyday life have become extremely difficult.
3 It is difficult to determine John's self-concept or self-image. The assumption is that he has little insight into his problems or the impact they will have on his life and social contacts.
4 John does not seem able to adapt to the physical and social changes in his life at the present.

Therapeutic self-care demand

Self-care agency

The self-care abilities (agency) of John have been determined. Essentially, John's self-care agency is non-functional, although there is potential for developing his existing abilities and cultivating new ones. He needs assistance with almost all aspects of care, as his existing system of care is inadequate to meet the demands placed upon him by his illness.

Self-care limitations

John has self-care limitations in most areas of his universal self-care requisites, and problems with developmental and health-deviation self-care requisites. In particular, there are physical restrictions which severely impair his ability to be self-caring. There are also psychological ones: he is experiencing mood changes which are interfering with his judgement in making essential self-care decisions. Communication is a problem. He is greatly frustrated by his difficulty in communication, and while he appears to understand what is being said to him, making his wishes known to others is proving difficult. John is also experiencing a knowledge deficit. It is assumed that he is not fully cognisant of his situation, its ramifications for his social and physical development, or the changes he must undergo to return to a familiar environment.

John has some specific knowledge deficits about his condition, such as the types of exercises required in order to improve his condition and to prevent complications, such as contractures. He is also unable to make sound judgements and decisions. His emotional lability makes it difficult for him to concentrate for any great length of time. He easily becomes frustrated and discouraged; this leads to demotivation. Without motivation it is unlikely that any plan of care or action towards self-care will be successful. Because of his fatigue and exhaustion, John does not have the energy necessary to sustain self-care behaviours for any great length of time.

John has a wide range of self-care deficits. He needs assistance in almost all areas of care from nursing and other staff during the period of his hospitalisation. This assistance is required not just to meet the self-care demands to live – that is, food and water – but also to prevent accidents and complications of his condition. The care offered to John is aimed at producing an environment that will foster his general development, but in particular the cultivation of new physical and social skills.

Resultant self-care demand

John's self-care demands have been calculated by examining his self-care abilities and self-care limitations. His condition suggests that there must be adjustments in his universal self-care requisites: specifically, he needs to achieve an early self-care ability to prevent accidents and further injury. Furthermore, action is necessary to avoid complications associated with a cerebrovascular accident, such as deep vein thrombosis as a result of prolonged immobility. In addition to these demands, John needs to modify his self-concept and to actively engage in preventive health-care behaviours.

PLANNING

Nursing actions

The nurses' role in caring for John involves compensating for his self-care inabilities and helping him to meet his universal self-care requisites. Nursing assistance is also required to support and protect him while allowing any existing abilities to be cultivated, and, wherever possible, fostering new ones (Tables 3.1 and 3.2).

Orem suggests that nurses can perform a wide range of activities to assist patients move towards a position where they can take a more active and decisive role in their care. The nature of John's situation suggests that, initially at least, a wholly compensatory nursing system will be required for his care, with the principal nursing actions being the performing of many care activities for him and, in general, acting on his behalf. Nursing actions will need to be aimed towards either acting or doing for John, or perhaps, in some situations, guiding or directing his own actions. However, he will be encouraged to help himself in any way possible. Additionally, psychological and spiritual support will be offered. It is important to emphasise that this range of nursing actions must take place in an appropriate environment. There must be times for quietness and rest, privacy, and activity. An important aspect of John's care plan is finding a suitable balance of environmental needs.

Nursing activities will be reviewed in response to John's progress in taking more responsibility for his own care. There may be a move away from nurses simply performing care for him, towards their offering more guidance and direction for him to perform some of his own self-care behaviours. Again, this nursing assistance must take place within an appropriate environment and with suitable psychological support.

Patient actions

John's role in his own care is both passive and active. Some self-care activities, such as managing eating and drinking, require his co-operation and assistance. The same can be said of encouraging communication and social interaction. However, activities such as exercises to increase flexibility and mobility in his right side are likely to be passive, in that he is unable to assist in them. A future goal might be to encourage John to use his left arm to exercise his right side. This could work if he understands why this is important

45

Table 3.1 *Assessment of John's universal self-care abilities and limitations*

Universal self-care requisites	Self-care abilities	Self-care limitations
The maintenance of a sufficient intake of air	Breathes without difficulty Coughs and deep-breathes spontaneously	Decreased mobility: potential for upper respiratory tract infection
The maintenance of a sufficient intake of water	Uses left arm/hand to hold glass Can direct hand to mouth accurately Can drink fluids but dribbles from right side of mouth	Right facial weakness Difficulty in swallowing Mobility: cannot obtain own fluids Requires prompting to drink: potential for dehydration
The maintenance of a sufficient intake of food	Can move left arm/hand to feed with assistance Can move hand to mouth Initiates swallowing	Dysphagia Poor appetite Requires prompting to eat: potential for malnutrition Mobility: cannot obtain own food
The provision of care associated with elimination processes and excrement	None	Cannot control voiding Cannot control bowel function Unaware of being incontinent Unable to manage hygiene of urino-genital and anal areas
The maintenance of a balance between activity and rest	Can rest and sleep for short periods only Uses left side to obtain a comfortable position	Difficulty sleeping: potential for fatigue/exhaustion Unable to turn self from side to side: potential for the development of pressure-area sores

Self-care requisite	Abilities	Problems
		Unable to walk without considerable assistance Unable to transfer self between bed and commode
The maintenance of a balance between solitude and social integration	Is able to indicate some wants and needs Recognises relations/friends/nursing staff Understands conversation from relatives Can understand nursing staff to assist in care where possible	Difficulty with speech: expressive aphasia Frustration/anger with communication difficulties Distances himself from family/friends and staff at times
The prevention of hazards to life, human functioning, and human well-being	Possesses pain sensation throughout body, but diminished sensation of right side Possesses vibration/touch sensation Has an acute sense of hearing	Poor coordination of movements Disorientation to day/date/time/place Visual disorder (hemianopia) Communication difficulties Diminished sensation
Normacy	Has limited communication skills Is able to gesture with left hand	Reduced communication, both verbal and non-verbal Reduced mobility Visual difficulties limit perception of the environment Altered self-concept and body image Altered self-esteem

Table 3.2 *Self- and nursing-action components of John's care*

Universal self-care requisites	Patient actions	Nursing actions
The maintenance of a sufficient intake of air	• Cough and deep-breathe • Expectorate	• Encourage coughing and deep-breathing • Monitor sputum for changes in colour and consistency • Assess respiratory adequacy (skin and nailbed colour)
The maintenance of a sufficient intake of water	• Use of left arm/hand for drinking • Drinking • Swallowing	• Encourage and assist with drinking as necessary • Ensure that fluids are in reach • Keep and maintain a fluid balance record • Observe for signs of dehydration
The maintenance of a sufficient intake of food	• Use of left arm when eating • Swallowing • Eating	• Assess for adequacy of swallowing • Ensure that food is presented in a manageable form • Assist with eating, as necessary • Keep and maintain a record of consumption • Supplement diet with vitamins/protein as necessary • Modify diet to prevent constipation
The provision of care associated with elimination processes and excrement		• Keep and maintain a record of urine output and bowel movements • Maintain hygiene in the perianal area
The maintenance of a balance between activity and rest	• Assist with mobility exercises • Assist with ambulation	• Provide an environment suitable for rest/quiet times, and one that will lessen frustration and anger • Ensure by using exercises that deformities are prevented

		• Provide assistance as necessary to other professional groups such as physiotherapists, speech therapists and occupational therapists
The maintenance of a balance between solitude and social integration	• Maintain channels of communication • Allow visits from friends	• Provide a suitable environment for social interaction • Provide a means of orientating John to his environment (e.g. calendar, clock, pictures of friends) • Provide aids for communication (e.g. picture/spell boards) • Ensure that nursing actions are consistent; establish a routine which can be flexible • Explain procedures and events carefully • Offer positive comment on actions achieved by John • Encourage him to meet other people
The prevention of hazards to life, human functioning, and human well-being	• Summon assistance before attempting to move	• Monitor vital signs and assess for changes in physical or psychological condition • Control environment to lessen the likelihood of accident or injury (e.g. use bed-rails at night)

Normalcy	• Maintain communication with staff and friends
	• Interact with others as appropriate
		• Encourage an environment where John can develop:
		  – self-esteem
		  – an improved body image
		  – a sense of trust in those around him
		  – ways to lessen the effects of anxiety and sense of loss
		  – understanding of his condition

and is motivated to carry it out. A routine needs to be established for care activities, to provide some consistency and orientation in his day.

John will be encouraged to participate in his own care at every possible opportunity, following suitable explanation. However, because of his fatigue, he must not be overworked. By encouraging participation, an opportunity will be provided to allow him to improve his existing ability and to develop new skills. Further, he can begin to take a greater interest in his own care.

The environment will be significant: a noisy or busy situation will decrease John's ability to concentrate. Additionally, he will need privacy when eliminating. It is important, too, to consider the timing of nursing interventions: when he is tired or upset, nursing or other professional staff interventions will need to be delayed whenever possible, until he has become more receptive to assistance.

EVALUATION

After two weeks on the acute medical ward, John has made some progress in managing the day-to-day necessities of living. Among the major difficulties are the psychological and emotional problems he has been experiencing. While attempts to orientate him through the use of clocks and calendars, are beginning to be successful – he can indicate on a calendar the day of the week – his emotional instability is a major cause for concern. He will still break down and cry at various times during the day without apparent precipitating cause. He has a short attention span, so that any attempt at patient education has to be kept short. Yet John needs to know something about his condition and why certain procedures are being performed. Following education sessions both with nursing staff and speech therapists aimed at improving his awareness of his situation, it remains difficult to determine just how much he has understood. Communication continues to be difficult despite intense intervention by the speech therapist.

John is not motivated to continue with ˥ any of the exercises or social activities on the ward. He gives up easily or tries to avoid them. He has begun to regain some ability to make decisions; he can, for example, indicate which clothes he wants to wear. However, most of the day-to-day decision-making processes, such as when to take a bath, still have to be initiated by nursing staff.

There has been relatively little improvement in John's physical condition. The aphasia and visual difficulty have shown little signs of improvement. Fortunately his cough and gag reflex have remained intact and prevented any aspiration. He can cough on demand and has so far avoided developing a chest infection. His blood pressure has decreased to 140/75 and his pulse is regular. Incontinence remains a problem, as does the resulting excoriation to his sacral area. Despite many attempts to encourage him to use a urinal he simply cannot: he doesn't know when he needs to void or have a bowel movement. He likes privacy, but even providing this has not helped him overcome elimination difficulties. In response to this, nursing staff are now instigating a regular programme of taking John to the toilet, to develop bladder and bowel habits and to keep his sacral area as clean and dry as possible.

His right-sided weakness remains a problem for mobility despite active physiotherapy and nursing interventions. No significant return in functioning has occurred and he has developed a marked right-sided inattention, despite efforts to remind him that he does have two arms and two legs. While he is able to support his weight on his left leg, he still requires two members o. staff to do any transferring from bed to chair or bath, and there remains the risk of accidental falls. Active physiotherapy continues, and following a case conference a decision has been made to offer John a wheelchair to encourage mobility. This would permit him to go outside to enjoy some fresh air and a change of environment. Provided that the wheelchair is presented in a positive light rather than as further proof of his disability, it may have a positive impact upon his psychological condition and motivate him to want to perform more activities for himself. His left arm is becoming more dexterous and the accuracy of hand–mouth activity is improving; there is less accidental spilling of food and drink. The occupational therapist has provided special rubber mats to prevent plates from moving on his tray, and this has given John a little more confidence and independence.

It is difficult to assess the degree to which John is managing the psychological and emotional impact of his condition. In particular, mainly due to communication problems, it is difficult to determine just how much he knows about his condition. This aspect of nursing care remains problematic. Although he has started to become a little more cooperative with hospital staff (particularly members of the physiotherapy department) he would much rather stay in bed if allowed to. However, exercises for arms and legs are done frequently during the day. He will often 'fight' against doing these, but most of the time allows others to help him. This could be interpreted as John

51

beginning to gain more insight into his condition. Determining the impact of the CVA on John's self-concept and body image is difficult. He has started to make some adaptations to his condition by using his left hand to eat and drink: this has begun to make his self-care activities more independent.

Summary

The initial care plan constructed for John has clearly not been completely successful in achieving all of its aims: it has not moved him to a position of being self-caring within the bounds of his abilities. This situation should not be viewed as a failure. Patients do respond to interventions in quite different ways, and after an initial period of 'stabilisation' of his immediate physical condition, rehabilitation has commenced. This, by its very nature, is a process of planning care, assessing patient outcomes, and often introducing new plans and new ideas for care.

There has been some improvement in John's condition, but many difficulties remain to be overcome. Nevertheless, the plan has moved John to a position where he is moving towards a situation of bodily functions which will be 'normal' for him, albeit slowly; where he is being encouraged to continue to grow and develop new skills; where further injuries have been prevented and rehabilitation has been commenced; and where some compensation has occurred for his disability (for example in the increasing use of his left hand). Many problems remain, including those of a physical nature, but especially that of promoting well-being. Determining John's feelings and opinions will be important for future progress, yet they remain a major challenge for nursing staff.

Postscript

A month later, John continues to show improvement in his coordination and movement. While not being able to walk unaided, he is willing to participate more in his care. Verbal communication remains a problem, but he is much less frustrated by this than before, and there appears to be less emotional turbulence. He now enjoys the visits from his friends and does his best to interact with them. Some problems, however, are still evident. In particular, he still lacks the ability to make judgements and take action with his own care. This situation remains a concern in the rehabilitation process and will affect the timeframe for his eventual discharge.

FOLLOW-UP WORK

Questions

1 The choice of nursing system for John was wholly compensatory. To what extent do you agree that this was appropriate? Could the care plan have been rewritten such that each universal self-care deficit was *individually* assessed as being wholly or partly compensatory or supportive/educative? Which universal requisites could have been considered either partly compensatory or supportive/educative?

2 It was very difficult to assess John's knowledge of his condition. What methods might you have used to determine how much he knew about his illness?

3 What are the problems involved in trying to assess patients when they are unable to communicate accurately and consistently with you, or when there is no one else to ask? How do you validate your findings?

4 Self-esteem and changes in body image are important issues for anyone who has suffered a health problem. Suggest ways in which these psychological aspects of care can be assessed. How would you work with John to improve his self-perception?

5 What other techniques could have been used to motivate John to participate in his own care? How important was the environment in determining the success of the care plan?

6 Incontinence was a persistent problem for John. What could be done to avoid the risk of urinary tract infection and excoriated sacral areas? How can the embarrassment of incontinence be minimised?

7 The problems John was experiencing with communication could have wider implications, extending to the giving of consent to treatment. If John needed to have a minor operation, what approach would you use to seek his consent? How would you determine the extent of his knowledge of his situation, of the need to have surgery and of the risks involved? How would you document your actions or findings?

Exercises

The following two exercises are designed to help you think about applying Orem's model in the care of your own patients. It is suggested that you work in small groups, perhaps of 6–8 people, with one of you making notes of your group's decisions. This will help you keep an accurate record of your findings. You may need to spend 20 – 30 minutes discussing your ideas with each other. Groups can then discuss their findings with each other.

Please use your tutor or facilitator to help clarify issues or to assist in 'brainstorming'. Remember that there are rarely 'correct' answers to any care-planning question. Use each other as resources, as well as Chapter 1 of this book. Some may wish to use Orem's own book as a source of information and guidance. Whatever source of information you use, please remember to think of your patient as a human being, and Orem's model simply as a means of guiding your data-collection and questioning, and providing a framework for giving and evaluating care.

Exercise 1

Consider an assessment you have recently made of a patient, either individually or in small groups. Put the assessment information you have gathered into the classification of universal, developmental and health-deviation self-care requisites suggested by Orem. For universal self-care requisites, allocate your data into the eight categories.

Consider the following issues. Were you able to assign your assessment data into the Orem classification scheme without difficulty? If not, what were the problems? How did you overcome them?

Exercise 2

In small groups, consider the plan of care suggested for John. What changes would you make to it if he was married and his wife was willing to help in his care? Consider the nature and quality of information available initially in assessing him, and how you would involve her in his care. Write down your ideas under the headings *Nursing actions*, *Patient's actions* and *Wife's actions*. Discuss your findings with your colleagues.

Activities

When he returns home John will face many problems. He is likely to have reduced coordination and muscle strength down one side of his body and will continue to experience perceptual and communication difficulties. This has important implications for him when managing self-care at home, especially in activities of daily living, communication and mobility.

Activity 1

Imagine that you find yourself in John's situation, having the use of only one of your hands. (You may find it helpful to put a sock on the hand with reduced mobility, to remind yourself not to use it.) During the course of a day, consider the difficulties in performing the following tasks:

- dressing/undressing;
- washing/bathing;
- meal preparation;
- toileting.

Share your experiences with your colleagues. What common problems did you encounter? How did you solve some of them?

Activity 2

A major concern for John will be to prevent hazards and accidents both in the home and outside. In groups of perhaps three or four, examine the dangers to mobility in your own neighbourhood. Consider aspects such as the following:

- The condition of pavements – are there broken paving slabs, or uneven or damaged surfaces?
- Are there kerb cuts in pavements to allow people to cross without having to step down into the road? (This is particularly important for wheelchairs.)
- Are pedestrian crossings conveniently available to allow people to cross roads safely?
- At pelican crossings, which are pedestrian-controlled, how long does the 'green man' stay illuminated, indicating that it is safe to cross? Is there enough time for an individual with impaired mobility to cross unhurriedly?
- Do roads and paths have adequate lighting?
- Evaluate access to public and other buildings. Are there stairs to climb to enter the library, post office or shops? Are doorbells and entryphones accessible?

Compare your findings with those of your colleagues. What common strengths and weaknesses have you identified in your physical environment?

Now that you have collected potentially valuable data about your community, do you plan to do anything with it? Could this information be used to bring about improvements? If so, how?

CHAPTER FOUR

Care study: living with diabetes mellitus

MARY

Mary is a 69-year-old woman who was diagnosed five years ago as having maturity-onset diabetes mellitus. She has lived by herself since the death of her husband some twenty years earlier. She had two children: Richard, now married with his own family, and a daughter, Anne, who died of a spinal tumour when she was eighteen. Richard lives in the same town as his mother, but the two of them rarely meet. Anne apparently excelled in all she did, but Richard could never live up to her achievements. He has, however, become a successful builder and provides a comfortable lifestyle for his family. Mary and Richard rarely talk with each other; this is a great source of sadness to her. She cannot understand why he stays away, or visits only when things are going seriously wrong. Has she done something wrong? Was it something she said? Richard is not keen to talk about his relationship with his mother, but did say on one occasion that it was 'tough competing with a dead sister'.

Mary lives in the Midlands, on the bottom floor of a block of council flats. This is important for her as she is finding stairs increasingly difficult to manage, becoming short of breath even after a couple of flights. She has no phone, but relies on her neighbours to relay phone messages to her sister who lives in the south of England, and occasionally to her son. Walking long distances is troublesome; fortunately there is a bus stop close to her flat and Mary makes an effort to go out every day, to collect a little shopping and to meet friends in the street. She cannot carry much as it hurts her arms and she has to stop and rest.

Mary was born in this town and has never been away for very long. Not having seen much of the country does not seem to bother

her; she is happy to meet the people with whom she went to school and has grown up over the years. She is staunchly independent, as are most of the older people in the town. While she enjoys the visits from her sister Patricia, she does not let her 'interfere' in her affairs, particularly where her son is concerned. Patricia has good relationships with Richard and with Mary, and works hard to bring them closer together. Unfortunately, this usually ends in antagonising both Mary and Richard.

Diabetic history

Mary suffers from maturity-onset diabetes, or non-insulin-dependent diabetes mellitus (NIDDM). This condition is usually associated with a lack of insulin or a change in insulin effectiveness. The first indications that problems were occuring became apparent five years ago when she saw her general practitioner on a routine visit for blood-pressure evaluation. She complained to him of having excessive thirst (polydipsia) and passing large amounts of urine (polyuria), of fatigue, of some occasional blurred vision, of tingling feelings in her hands and feet, and of an intense irritation in her perineum (puritis). The doctor performed a urinalysis and obtained a grossly elevated urine-sugar result.

Following further medical and laboratory examination as an in-patient at the local District General Hospital, Mary was formally diagnosed as having maturity-onset diabetes mellitus. Mary's doctor explained to her the cause of diabetes and the effects it might have on her. He outlined the possible causes of Mary's diabetes, which include inadequate amounts of insulin being produced, insulin somehow being made ineffective before it can take effect, insulin release not being in phase with dietary intake, or a decrease in receptor cells (Porth 1986, p.632).

He also told her that while maturity-onset diabetes can generally be controlled by diet, it is a condition which can lead to serious chronic complications including altered sensation in her hands and feet (neuropathies), changes in vision (retinopathies), vascular complications, infections, and damage to the kidneys (nephropathies). Mary appeared to have the beginnings of some of these problems.

Whilst she was being evaluated in the diabetic unit, a considerable amount of time was spent explaining to Mary the relationship between diabetes, diet and changes in lifestyle, particularly the need to have regular meals and the type and quantity of foods which should be eaten. Details were given about the way foods can be substituted for each other to provide a suitable diabetic diet. Information was also given about the care which must be given to her extremities, in particular in avoiding injury to her hands and feet. She was advised that she should notify her GP if she developed a cold, a cough or the flu; Mary appeared to understand this advice. Mary's GP also asked the district nurse when she was in the vicinity to see how Mary was managing.

ASSESSMENT

Today, Mary received an unfortunate injury at home when she slipped on the carpet while making tea and spilled boiling water on her legs. After being taken to the local accident and emergency unit for treatment of scalds which fortunately were not too severe, she has been admitted to the diabetic assessment unit. This move is considered necessary as her blood-sugar is grossly elevated. While this could be a reaction to the injury, it is considered prudent to evaluate more closely Mary's management of her diabetes. On arrival, following an orientation to the unit, she is assessed by the nursing staff.

Universal self-care requisites

Mary has a sharp mind and is able to recall in vivid detail the events of her life. It is clear, however, that her short-term memory is not always accurate. She realises this, and with a wry smile says, 'I know you think I'm dotty, but I'm as sane as you are.' She wears glasses to help her read but complains of occasional blurred vision. This worries her because there are times when she cannot see the number of the bus as it approaches. Sometimes she misses the one that stops close to her house: she then has to wait for another or walk home, a walk she finds increasingly tiring. She does not mention any other changes in her health, other than to complain of 'pins and needles in my hands and feet'.

She is able to breathe regularly and there is no audible wheezing. She admits that at times she has to 'stop and catch my breath for a while' when out walking. This is due, she claims, to 'getting on a bit in years' and 'having to lose a pound or two in weight'. In fact, Mary has been putting on weight over the past couple of years. She knows this is a problem and is concerned that her doctor will find out and become upset with her. She also smokes cigarettes – not many, she claims, but there are tobacco stains on her fingers.

She is good at keeping her appointments with the doctor, and while not knowledgeable about recent dietary suggestions to avoid heart disease and control diabetes, she 'does as she's told'. Basically, she has complete faith in her doctor.

Along with the rise in weight has been noted an increase in her blood pressure, and Mary is being treated for this. She takes 'two little green pills' every day for blood-pressure control. The reason for the blood-pressure increase is not precisely known, but it has been suggested that her weight is a contributing factor.

Managing her diabetic diet is important, and she keeps some of the information given to her by the district nurse in her purse. She is not, however, a slave to it. 'A little bit of what you fancy does you good', she says, and freely admits to eating chocolate bars. She also likes more than the occasional glass of sherry. These dietary supplements do not seem to concern her, and she does not seem aware of the possible health implications of her behaviour.

Mary likes routine, particularly when going to bed and getting up in the mornings. She has had no difficulty sleeping until recently, and has never taken any sleeping pills. Sleeping can be a problem for her now as a bypass to keep traffic away from the town has recently been built close to her house and the noise of the large lorries sometimes keeps her awake. Usually, however, she sleeps soundly, and denies having shortness of breath at night.

During the days she likes to get out, provided the weather is fine. Since the death of her husband she does not like staying inside the house by herself. Sometimes in the street she meets people she knows, and may stop to speak with them. Few are ever invited back to her flat. 'Don't want them nosing in my stuff', she will say, not wanting other people to know too much about her. She does, however, have morning coffee with one particular woman who lives not far away, whom she has known for many years. They like to reminisce about the 'old days' and catch up on the local town gossip. Her friend will sometimes ask about Richard, but Mary quickly changes the subject.

Developmental and health-deviation self-care requisites

Assessment of developmental and health-deviation self-care requisites for the diabetic patient can be guided by the work of Fitzgerald (1980). She suggests the following headings for consideration.

Impact of diagnosis

Following discussions with Mary, it appears that the diagnosis of diabetes is causing her no great distress. She does not see the condition as a 'disabling' one; it carries no particular stigma for her, although she does not advertise the fact that she is diabetic.

Experience with illness

Nobody in Mary's family has previously been affected by diabetes; this perhaps accounts for the apparent absence of stigma. It seems that in the first few months of being diagnosed as diabetic, Mary had no particularly poor experiences; she lived her life as she always had done, apart from trying to manage changes in diet, taking rest periods more frequently, and testing her urine. In more recent times, however, there have been some increasing difficulties with sensation and with the resultant impact on her fine motor movements, presumably due to the diabetes. Her walking has also been affected by increasing shortness of breath on exercise. This might be due to the diabetes, or to her weight increase.

Motivation

Mary is obviously motivated to continue to care for herself. Her attention to the diabetic condition and to keeping regular appointments with the doctor is evidence of this. However, although she is motivated to keep her 'independence' there are obvious problems with her knowledge of the diabetic condition and the dietary management of this condition.

Energy and movement

In order for an individual to manage a diabetic condition Backscheider (1974) has suggested that the following conditions must be considered:

Physical Mary must be able to manage the physical aspects of her own care and the diabetes. This will include not only the dexterity to manage regular urine-testing, but also the ability to manage obtaining a suitable diet and the washing and care of extremities. She is having some ocular problems and the tingling in her fingers appears

61

to be more noticeable. For the most part, however, Mary does seem to be able to manage the physical aspects of caring.

Mental   Individuals must have the appropriate cognitive skills to be able to manage their condition. Mary, despite having had explained to her the importance of diet, exercise and the avoidance of activities likely to aggravate her condition, still chooses to smoke and drink. While this in itself is not the major issue, the fact that Mary does not seem to realise the potential harm she is doing to herself is an important consideration. She does not seem fully aware of the care she must adopt to prevent or minimise further damage to her health.

Motivational   Mary is motivated to look after herself. This may in part be because of her desire to remain independent, or because she is concerned that if she fails to do so her doctor will be angry with her. Whatever the reasons, it is clear from her behaviour that Mary is motivated to manage her own care. Yet there appears to be conflict between her desire to look after herself and her desire to smoke and to eat 'unwisely' for her condition.

Impact on daily life

Until recently Mary has had few problems with her daily living routine. However, increasing shortness of breath on walking and climbing stairs has caused Mary some discomfort and annoyance; this is affecting her quality of life. As this is coupled with the difficulties she has had in seeing bus numbers and in manipulating small objects, Mary is beginning to realise that she needs help.

Duration of diabetes

Clearly, the duration of the diabetes is beginning to have an impact on Mary's life. She is now becoming much more aware of the changes which are occurring to her. She wants to overcome these.

Eating habits

Diet is important to the management of diabetes, and Mary does realise this. While she possesses details of the need for a diabetic diet and the exchange list for foods, she is fairly 'creative' with her diet. Chocolate and alcohol need to be taken strictly in moderation.

PLANNING

Self-care agency

Mary does have some self-care ability; she knows, for example, something about diabetes, although there are obvious limitations in that knowledge. She has been taught about the management of diabetes, she can recall aspects of management and, for the most part, she has the motor skills to look after herself and perform BM stick testing. She has also, to some degree, integrated her condition into everyday life: she goes out, she meets people, and she manages important aspects of self-care such as the provision of food.

Self-care limitations

Nevertheless, self-care limitations are evident. An important observation is that Mary has a limited knowledge of her condition. While she is aware of the general nature of her condition ('too much sugar in my urine'), there is a knowledge deficit about diet and the management of symptoms and lifestyle. She is not able, for example, to make sensible substitutions as part of her diabetic diet. This goes beyond the 'a little bit of what you fancy does you good' argument, where all people want some variety in their dietary routines. Missing meals and then overeating to compensate is not appropriate for her condition. She is also not sure about what to do if she became unwell. Should she visit the doctor or wait a while?

At times, when her blood-sugar is high, she is unable to think clearly and make sound judgements about self-care. Combined with her frequent bouts of fatigue there are days when she cannot, or does not, go out. There are also some physical limitations; ocular changes and some loss of sensation in her hand make fine movement and coordination difficult. This is particularly important when it comes to accurate urine-testing. She is not always able to do this with the skill and accuracy necessary to obtain consistent results.

Developmentally, the impact of being diagnosed as diabetic does not appear to have caused Mary a great deal of distress. While she is still able to pursue her life fairly independently she appears to be content. Fortunately there have been no sudden changes; Mary's condition results in the insidious development of problems which so far, physically at least, she is coping with.

Mary appears to be able to manage some of the health-deviation self-care requisites associated with being diabetic. She has been seeking advice from nursing staff and her GP as well as maintaining her regular appointments with her doctor. Mary is aware of some of the side-effects of the condition; she is becoming more aware of these as her condition changes. Generally she is compliant as far as appointment-keeping is concerned, but following the general guidelines of diabetic dietary management is not easy for her. Her reluctance to stop smoking and her frequent indulgence in sweet food may be having a direct adverse effect on her health. Mary has begun to manage the unpleasant impact of diabetes; she is having to plan her shopping trips more carefully. However, there are still several dangers in the home which need to be attended to; loose carpets on the floors coupled with failing vision could lead to a fall and subsequent injury. While Mary is managing many aspects of her condition, there is concern about the educational aspects of diabetic management which will need nursing intervention.

Therapeutic self-care demand

Based upon the above assessment, the following care plan is suggested.

Universal self-care requisites

1 Maintain an adequate intake of air:
 • Prevent further damage to lungs by stopping smoking.
2 Maintain a sufficient intake of food:
 • Ensure that Mary's diet is appropriate for her diabetic condition.
 • Reinforce the need to adhere to the diet.
 • Stress the importance of having meals at regular intervals.
3 Maintain a sufficient intake of fluids:
 • Drink several glasses of fluids throughout the day.
 • If juices are used, ensure that they are appropriate for a diabetic person.
 • Avoid alcohol if possible.
4 Care associated with elimination:
 • To avoid constipation, aim to increase the fibre in the diet.
 • Ensure a sufficient fluid intake.
 • Ensure that perianal areas are kept clean by frequent washing/ bathing

5 Maintain a balance between rest and activity:
- Ensure sufficient sleep during the night.
- Ensure rest breaks throughout the day.

6 Maintain a balance between solitude and social interaction:
- Encourage Mary to continue to meet her friends.
- Recognise her need for privacy and solitude.

7 Prevent hazards:
- Take particular care with extremities; avoid injury if possible.
- Ensure that spectacles are worn and are appropriate for her.
- Educate Mary to carry information at all times about being a diabetic.
- Consider obtaining a bracelet or necklace warning of a diabetic condition.
- Develop Mary's awareness of early signs of low blood-sugar.
- Examine the environment for potential hazards, e.g. poorly fitting carpets.

8 Normacy:
- Mary needs to move towards the integration into everyday life of being a diabetic.
- She needs to be aware of physical limitations due to advancing years but not let these stop her enjoying life.
- She should live life to the full, but within the limitations of being a diabetic.

Developmental self-care requisites

1 Maintain Mary's responsibility for her own care.
2 Ensure that others, particulary friends, are aware of her diabetic condition.
3 Try to involve her son in the management of her diabetes.

Health-deviation self-care requisites

1 Ensure that Mary can recognise when she might be developing hyperglycaemia.
2 Ensure that she is aware of the action that should be taken if any symptoms of hyperglycaemia should develop.
3 Develop an awareness of the impact of illness or changes in health on a diabetic person.
4 Educate Mary to obtain prompt assistance if illness develops.
5 Continue with regularly timed health evaluations.
6 Mary needs to continue keeping appointments when scheduled.

7 She needs to develop routines in her life which involve regular meals, energy expenditure and self-monitoring of urine-sugar.

Nursing system

A supportive/educative nursing system has been developed for Mary. While she is able to meet many aspects of her care there are some specific areas, particularly educational, with which she requires assistance. An important aspect of this system is the negotiation of roles that Mary and nursing staff will adopt. Mary is independent in many things and an over-intrusive care plan might lead to her deciding not to participate in improving her self-care abilities.

Following discussions, Mary has agreed to adopt a participatory role in her care. In particular, she will talk to the dietitian and will spend time with the nurse who is responsible for the diabetic management of patients. In addition, she has agreed to participate in diabetic education classes: this will involve going to classes with other diabetic people to learn more about their condition, and to share experiences. However, there will also be some individual sessions.

In order to improve existing self-care abilities and develop new ones, the following agreement is reached between Mary and nursing staff about individual responsibilities.

Mary's involvement

Mary will:

- perform and record accurately urine glucose-testing twice daily;
- plan a menu for meals of two days at a time;
- prepare food according to the menu and eat the food at regular times during the day;
  - try not to eat between meals;
  - avoid alcoholic beverages;
  - reduce (preferably stop) smoking;
  - plan to take rest breaks during the day;
  - plan shopping trips to coincide with the bus service, when possible;
  - continue to wear spectacles;
  - manage personal hygiene.

Nursing responsibility

Nursing staff will:

- provide some initial assistance in performing urine-sugar analysis;
- evaluate Mary's urinalysis technique;
- reinforce dietary information;
- assist in the planning of meals and rest periods;
- review the importance of good personal hygiene and the avoidance of injuries;
- review the warning signs of elevated glucose levels;
- review the management of any 'unusual' physical sensations possibly associated with an elevated glucose level.

IMPLEMENTATION

Small-group and individual education sessions are used with Mary to support her existing behaviours and knowledge, and to develop these. An education plan has been devised for Mary which outlines all the key aspects of personal care, including care to extremities when one has diabetes. This involves Mary being shown appropriate methods for looking after her skin and nails. This is further supplemented by the use of written material prepared by hospital staff and by the British Diabetic Association. Mary is encouraged to ask questions throughout the sessions. Later she is asked to demonstrate key aspects of care in the presence of nursing staff. A similar approach is used by the dietitian, who stresses the importance of maintaining a suitable diet to ensure good general nutrition as well as one that is appropriate for Mary's diabetic condition. Emphasis is placed upon understanding the principles of dietary management of diabetes, in particular which foods can be eaten as part of the diet and which should be avoided. Variety is important, and the dietitian advises Mary that there is now a range of confectionery suitable for diabetic patients which she could safely eat; this can, however, be quite expensive. Nursing staff concentrate their supporting and teaching roles on helping Mary to understand the importance of being aware of her condition, and alert her to the feelings she may experience if her blood-sugar level changes.

Mary is also invited to participate in some small-group sessions where other people with similar conditions are asked to share some of their experiences of being diabetic. Participants take time to introduce themselves and are encouraged to discuss any aspect of their lives related to diabetes which they feel comfortable discussing.

A particular focus of the group is on diet; how do others deal with the temptation to eat unsuitable foods and luxuries? How do they ensure that their lives can be lived fully and that their diabetes does not become a 'disabling condition'?

EVALUATION

The time spent with Mary has made some impact upon her daily life and her ability to be self-caring. Following discharge from hospital and follow-up from community nursing staff, there appear to have been some noticeable changes in Mary's behaviour. She is much more aware of the dietary management of diabetes and can now prepare a suitable menu when asked by the district nurse to do so. It is rather too soon to see how Mary deals with the urges she has for alcohol and tobacco, but at least she is now fully aware of the possible impact of these on her health.

She is much more careful in looking after her skin, using only the mildest of soaps and taking more time to dry herself. Also, she has become more comfortable wearing her spectacles. Many aspects of her home environment, however, have not changed. There are still some dangerously loose carpets on the floor, and she still feels unable to ask her son for help. Many of the issues in Mary's daily living clearly cannot be addressed by nursing intervention. The volume of traffic on the roads, for example, has not changed. Instead Mary adjusts her sleeping patterns so that she is in bed when the traffic noise is least.

In general, it appears that Mary is coming to terms with the developmental and health-deviation self-care demands placed upon her. She still tries to live as full a life as possible, not being unduly hindered in living the way she wants to. She is demonstrating many of the behaviours which are important for the self-management of diabetes. She is compliant with medical and nursing requests, and has shown that she can adapt to the changes she has undergone due to diabetes. Self-image has always been difficult to assess with Mary, and this aspect of her life remains an enigma.

Regrettably, the wish to further involve family and friends to help Mary live with her condition has not been successful. This is much in keeping with her participation in the group sessions held at the clinic, where she was uncomfortable and obviously unable or unwilling to express her feelings in public. Nevertheless, Mary is living a fulfilled life in her own terms, now aware of the self-care behaviours she must continue if she is to avoid aggravating her diabetic condition.

FOLLOW-UP WORK

Questions

The following questions could be answered individually or used as group exercises. As with other care studies, small groups of 6–8 people could be used to address the issues which follow; 20–30 minutes' discussion on each should be sufficient. Remember to nominate a note-taker. Use your tutor or facilitator to help you in discussions: their role is particularly important if you feel that you cannot make any progress with an issue and are at an impasse.

1 Mary seemed to have a failing memory for some short-term events. What special problems does this pose when assessing her? How might this fact influence Mary's care?
2 What is the health-education role for nursing? How might this be reflected in a patient's care plan? Would you have used a different approach in managing Mary's care?
3 For patient education to take place there must be motivation and a sense of readiness to learn. How can this motivation and readiness be assessed? Was Mary ready to learn? Explain.
4 Much of Mary's care was supportive/educative. This suggests that nursing staff would allow her to take her own decisions and be as participative as possible in her own care. What factors in a patient are important to consider before adopting a supportive/educative nursing system? Would you have adopted this nursing system with Mary? Explain.
5 One of the nursing interventions adopted with Mary was the use of small groups. What factors do you think should be present in a patient before using this approach? Why was it unsuccessful with Mary? What other methods could have been used?
6 Patient education is central to Mary's care. What methods could be adopted to ensure that Mary had understood the information given to her? Using a longer-term perspective, would those same methods be appropriate six months later?
7 Mary clearly liked to eat and drink things she probably should not. What would you say to Mary if you found her eating small quantities of chocolate? On a wider issue, you are likely to encounter many patients who are unwell and who continue to

follow practices which probably should be curtailed, for example smoking. What is your general reaction to this situation? How do you plan to manage it?

Activities

Mary, when she returns home, will need to ensure that she maintains her current circle of friends; it will be important for her to maintain a balance between activity and rest and between solitude and social integration.

Activity 1

In groups of three or four go into your community and investigate the services or activities which are available for older people. In particular, consider the following:

- Where do the elderly meet – in the pub, in a café, on a park bench?
- What role does the library have for some elderly people? (Remember that during winter these are often warm places; there can be free book loans, and large-print books are often available.)
- Are there any lunch clubs for the elderly in your area? What role do you think these play in maintaining social contacts?
- Consider transportation needs. Is there a frequent and reliable bus service? Is there special assistance available to those who need it? Are concessionary fares available and well publicised?

Activity 2

Mary continues to have sensory and perceptual difficulties, in particular loss of sensation in her hands and altered vision. These will be a concern for her as she must continue to avoid hazards and injury. Try the following, to simulate some of Mary's problems:

1 Wear socks on both hands and try tying your shoes, buttoning a shirt or blouse, or sorting small change.
2 Cover your eyes with different thicknesses and/or colours of plastics and try the following activities:
   - Write a letter to somebody.
   - Use the telephone.
   - Use the lift. Can you determine which floor you are on?

70

- Try catching a bus. How close do you have to be before you can read its number?

What advice would you offer people at discharge if they were experiencing sensory and perceptual difficulties? As regards the home in particular, what advice would you give to Mary on managing the temperature of hot water or of radiators?

CHAPTER FIVE

Care study: general surgical care

JILL

Jill is an ambitious 56-year-old woman, who has recently been promoted to branch manager of a local bank. This has put a great deal of stress on her, with long hours and frequent meetings and conferences. She has since had difficulty in establishing a daily routine for living; her eating habits in particular have been disrupted because of the large number of working lunches she must attend.

Jill and her husband Ian live confortably in a spacious house in the countryside. They have been married for over twenty years; Ian has always been very supportive of his wife's activities and professional ambitions, and they now feel they are beginning to see the rewards for all their efforts at work.

While Jill has been in good health for most of her life, over the past couple of years she has begun experiencing gastrointestinal pain. An examination at the local hospital revealed that she has cholecystitis. She has been treated conservatively by the use of a fat-reduction diet; this has been increasingly difficult to adhere to, however, because of her job and lifestyle. She has also been putting on weight.

More recently the intensity of Jill's pain has increased. Typically she experiences a sharp pain in the right upper quadrant of her abdomen, sometimes radiating to her right shoulder. This comes on quite suddenly and can last for hours. She sometimes breaks out in sweats, feels nauseous and vomits. This, she has observed, coincides with times when she has not complied with her diet and has eaten a large fatty meal. Coupled with this has been frequent indigestion, belching and flatulence. Occasionally she finds breathing difficult because of increased pain on inspiration; this causes her considerable anxiety. She has not, however, developed any of the more severe symptoms of cholecystitis, such as becoming jaundiced or passing clay-coloured stools.

Pathophysiology of cholecystitis

Cholecystitis is an inflammation of the gall bladder which can take the form of a chronic or an acute condition. It is also possible to have an acute attack superimposed upon a chronic one. Acute cholecystitis is almost always associated with an obstruction to the flow of bile. With this obstruction there is often inflammation of the gall bladder, believed to be caused by the chemical irritation of concentrated bile (Porth 1986). The gall bladder is often distended and may be the site of a bacterial infection resulting in fever and high white blood cell counts.

Management of cholecystitis

Jill is currently being treated in a conservative manner for cholescystitis by the use of a low-fat diet. The rationale for using this approach is firstly that reducing fat intake reduces gall bladder contractility and thus avoids pain, and secondly that a decrease in fat intake reduces the need for bile in the absence (or reduction) of gall bladder function (Billings and Stokes 1987). Several variations on a fat-restricted diet exist, but Table 5.1 indicates which foods Jill is encouraged to eat and which are to be avoided.

Table 5.1 *Low-fat diet suited to cholecystitis*

Allowed foods	Suggestions
Meat and egs	Lean meat, eggs limited to three per week
Milk	Skimmed milk
Fruits and vegetables	All accept avocado
Bread and cereals	All except hot breads

The following foods should be avoided: whole milk, ice cream, butter, cheese, chocolate, gravies and sauces, fried foods, potato crisps, fish soaked in oil, pork, mayonnaise, and lunch meats.

Jill is an intelligent and articulate person, and understands the link between diet and her condition, but she is experiencing some

73

personal and professional conflict. She believes that to continue to advance in her profession and to develop personally, she must continue to attend meetings where food and drink are at the centre of events. While some of these allow her to keep to the diet, most do not. Jill does want to be healthy and to lose weight, but at present does not have her life ordered such that she can reconcile these competing demands.

Over the past month, the frequency and intensity of painful episodes has been increasing. Following discussions with her physician and surgeon, it has been agreed that she should come into hospital and have her gall bladder removed (a cholescystectomy).

ASSESSMENT

Jill is admitted to her local hospital for surgery. Following a brief orientation to staff and the unit, she is assessed by her primary nurse using Orem's model as a framework.

Jill is fully alert and orientated when initially assessed by the nursing staff. She is experiencing no immediate physical problems or distress. Her initial vital sign readings are as shown in Table 5.2:

Table 5.2 *Jill's vital signs on assessment*

Vital sign	Value
Blood pressure	120/70
Pulse	80 and regular
Respiratory rate	18; no audible wheezing
Temperature	98.8° F
Blood measurements	Within normal limits, but low prothombin time

She is very cooperative and keen to find out more about her condition and what will happen over the next few days. Table 5.3 is a summary of the assessment made of Jill's condition. The primary nurse has decided to use Orem's framework in a flexible way more accurately to describe and analyse Jill's condition. The nurse, when collecting information from Jill, feels that the universal and developmental self-care requisites can be used in the way suggested by

Orem, but that it will be helpful to merge some of the health-deviation self-care requisites.

Additionally, it is important to consider Jill's current self-care abilities and her self-care deficits. Jill is to undergo an operation, which may put additional demands on her. Attention must therefore be given to *potential* self-care deficits that Jill may experience; these will be important in planning her care.

PLANNING

The care which Jill's primary nurse has identified for her is presented in Table 5.3. This care has been based upon the previous health assessment.

After assessing Jill's actual and potential self-care deficits, a decision must be taken about the nature of the nursing care to be given to her. Many aspects of her care will require the nurse actually to 'do' things for her, particularly when she returns from the recovery room. The nurse and the patient must together enter into a system of care in which some aspects are wholly compensatory; other aspects, though, will require a cooperative effort (the system is then partially compensatory), and some will require the nurse to support Jill's self-care and to be a source of information and an educator (when the system is supportive/educative).

Table 5.3 summarises the care plan suggested for Jill. It identifies those actions she will attempt to perform herself and those in which nursing staff will assist. The nature of the interaction between Jill and nursing staff is indicated in the 'Method of care' column. As with all care planning, there needs to be some timeframe established during which the outcomes of care are to be achieved. Initially this is set as the second day. However, it is expected that Jill will achieve many of the identified self-care actions soon after returning to her unit.

SURGERY

Preparation for surgery

Jill has come into hospital the day before surgery. During the evening of her admision, an assessment is made of her current condition, and the nursing staff spend time with her talking about the operation and the experiences she is likely to have. Jill finds this time particularly useful in reducing her feelings of stress. The

Table 5.3 *Summary of Jill's care plan*

Universal self-care requisites	Self-care abilities	Self-care deficits	Potential self-care deficits	Self-care actions	Nursing actions	Method of care
Maintain intake of air	Able to manage respiratory needs most of the time without assistance. When not in pain can cough and deep-breathe	When having right epigastric pain, breathing becomes difficult. Not always able to know more about splinting painful area when breathing and coughing. Becomes quite anxious when having pain which compromises breathing; needs to know more about anxiety-reduction techniques.	Following surgery there is a risk of further respiratory compromise because of incision/drains. Pain on deep-breathing may hinder coughing. There is the potential for infection or atelectasis because of immobility and failure to expand lungs fully periodically. Will require analgesia during periods of intense pain.	• Will ask for analgesia when needed • Will notify nurse if breathing becomes difficult or painful • Will learn to use a splinting technique to breathe/cough if there is pain • Will learn relaxation techniques during periods of pain	• Educate Jill about how to cough and deep-breathe while holding her incisional site • Recognise the need for analgesia • Position in bed to promote lung expansion; encourage mobility as soon as possible • Monitor sputum colour and texture • Observe Jill's colour • Observe and record respiratory rate	• Act for • Guide/direct • Educate
Maintain intake of fluids	Able to manage own fluid requirements when not nauseous or vomiting.	Unable to manage daily fluid requirements when nauseous or vomiting.	Following surgery there is the potential for fluid loss (including blood). This may affect blood pressure. There may be the need for intravenous fluid replacement. There is also the potential for electrolyte imbalance due to fluid loss or alterations in nutritional status.	• Communicate with nursing staff if nausea present • If permitted water, swallow only small amounts to begin with • Learn the purpose/action of the nasogastric tube (if required) • Notify the nurse if great thirst develops • Manage own mouth care soon after surgery	• Monitor patient for nausea/vomiting • Maintain an accurate fluid balance record • Offer fluids when bowel sounds heard • Care to mouth and oral mucosa (immediately post-operatively) • Monitor blood pressure/pulse at least hourly • Monitor output from any drains immediately post-operatively, then hourly	• Guide/direct • Support • Educate
Maintain intake of food	Physically and mentally able to understand the prescribed dietary intake. Can prepare own meals, and read guidelines on diet restrictions for the person with cholecystitis. Intellectually able to understand the purpose of the dietary restrictions	Seems to be unsure of what foods constitute a fat-restricted diet. Appears to like many foods which should be limited, and is unable to resist the temptation to eat these. During times of nausea and vomiting patient has not been able to eat.	Patient will not be able to eat or drink immediately following surgery. There may be a nasogastric tube in place. There is the potential for malnourishment if patient is not able to resume eating soon after surgery. Intravenous nutrients may be required. Jill will have to be prepared psychologically for this.	• Alert nursing staff if nausea or vomiting occurs • Let nursing staff know if feelings of hunger develop • Acquire information about the need for food restrictions following surgery	• Monitor gastrointestinal function • Offer anti-emetics if appropriate • Support patient by advising that gut motility often takes several hours to return after surgery, and that the nasogastric tube (if required) will help prevent gastric distension • Advise that this is quite 'normal' after an operation	• Guide/direct • Support • Educate

Need	Assessment	Potential problem	Patient goals	Nursing interventions	Nurse role
				• Monitor for signs of bleeding or excessive bruising	• Support • Educate
Manage elimination	Able to manage this need.	Potential for fat-soluble vitamin deficiency, particularly K (implications for blood coagulation). Potential for constipation following surgery because of immobility and possible fluid imbalance. Potential for difficulty in urinating following surgery.	• Notify nursing staff if bowel movement occurs or flatulence • Notify staff when the urge to void occurs	• Alert patient to the possibility of constipation following surgery • Mobilise the patient as soon as possible after surgery • Alert and remind Jill that urination and defecation may be difficult post-operatively	• Support • Educate
Balance activity and rest	Has been able to participate in all her usual activities, for example walking the dog. Sometimes having a restful night has been difficult. Following eating fatty foods pain has resulted which has caused restless nights. She has become quite fatigued	Following surgery, pain may continue to cause restlessness and difficulty sleeping. There is also the problem of being in an unfamiliar ward environment with noise and light preventing undisturbed rest. Vital signs may need to be taken during the night. Activity may be restricted immediately after surgery because of pain, intravenous therapy and surgical drains. This restriction should be short-lived.	• Recognise the need to have periods of rest • Try to rest/sleep during quieter times on the ward • Recognise the importance of activity and mobility as part of post-operative recovery • Plan to exercise as much as possible • Anticipate the need for assistance when first mobilising	• Plan nursing activities to permit the maximum opportunity for rest • Build in times for mobility/exercise • Anticipate the need to offer analgesia prior to exercise in the first few hours (or days) post-operatively • Recognise the need to take Jill's existing fatigue into account when arranging exercise • Observe for the development of pressure sores if patient is in bed for long periods	• Guide/direct • Support • Educate
Balance solitude and social interaction	Maintains close relationships with family and friends, but enjoys time by herself.	Tiredness may be exacerbated by surgery and the nature of the hospital environment. May become increasingly tired and fall asleep throughout the day, including visiting times. May become intolerant of nursing interventions and relatives/friends.	• Plan for quieter times during the day (solitude if necessary) to rest • Continue to interact with family and friends • Indicate when she is tired/fatigued	• Try to plan nursing activities to take into account the patient's wishes for time by herself • Monitor how tired Jill becomes around visiting times • Perhaps discuss with relatives the need to consider how long they stay with Jill in the evenings	• Support • Educate
Prevent hazards to life, well-being, and functioning:	Intellectually and physically able to prevent hazards to life if aware of them. Life-style problems and stress-management difficulties.	Will require continued adherence to fat-restricted diet, and other weight-loss strategies.	• Identify key food products which should be reduced/avoided on a fat-reduction diet	• Allow Jill the opportunity to discuss her lifestyle and its implications for her health (in a	• Support • Educate

Table 5.3 (cont'd) Summary of Jill's care plan

Universal self-care requisites	Self-care abilities	Self-care deficits	Potential self-care deficits	Self-care actions	Nursing actions	Method of care
1 Lack of understanding of the importance of diet of diet 2 Weight reduction	Aware of the importance of keeping to a fat-reduction diet. Aware of the importance of losing weight and in particular to her present condition.	Has a busy life, is often unable to manage time well enough to plan meals properly; eats at irregular times. Also has many business lunches where there is social pressure to eat.		• Consider lifestyle, and identify ways in which a change in diet (fat-restricted) can be incorporated into it • Consider ways of weight reduction with nurses and the dietitian	non-judgemental manner) • Discuss with Jill the importance of weight loss as part of her overall recovery from an operation • Discuss ways Jill might continue to be active in her profession yet still consider her health • Emphasise the importance of diet to Jill's future health following surgery • Ensure Jill meets with the dietitian	• Support • Educate
Promote normalcy; develop and maintain a realistic self-concept	An intelligent person who communicates her concerns, problems and aspirations well. She appears to have a realistic self-concept. She realises that she needs to lose weight, yet does not allow her physical appearance to interfere with her social relationships.	Appears not to have any obvious self-care problems related to self-concept.	Unsure of the impact of surgery or self-concept on body image.	• Continue to be self-confident in personal and professional activities following surgery • Continue to have a realistic self-concept while attempting to manage a change in diet and eating behaviours • Verbalise concerns about surgery and life after the operation	• Support and reinforce the need to incorporate dietary changes into lifestyle • Be a source of information or resource to Jill • Allow time for Jill to talk through her ideas of managing future change	• Support • Educate

Developmental self-care requisites	Self-care abilities	Self-care deficits	Potential self-care deficits	Self-care actions	Nursing actions	Method of care
Maintain lifestyle that promotes maturation	Jill has sufficient resources to maintain a high quality of life and to develop her interests. She has many leisure activities and gains great pleasures from them. She has many plans for the future, both in terms of	She has some concerns about the impact of her condition on her abilities to meet her personal and professional ambitions. She is unsure of the impact of surgery on her life, particularly her personal and professional development.	Jill may believe that the operation will resolve her dilemmas and conflicts. Surgery will not do this.	• Discuss concern about her professional and personal development following surgery • Indicate some of the strategies she might adopt in returning to work and interacting with her colleagues • Discuss some of the lifestyle	• Be a source of information about diet, in conjunction with dietary staff • Provide an environment where Jill feels comfortable talking about change • Be supportive of Jill's needs and drives	• Support • Educate

Health-care deviation self-care requisites	Self-care abilities	Self-care deficits	Potential self-care deficits	Self-care actions	Nursing actions	Method of care
	professional and personal development, in particular her desire to see as much of the world as possible.			changes she must make in order to move towards a more healthy state, e.g. weight loss and a fat-restricted diet	• Provide reassurance that Jill can return to a healthy state and maintain it	
Seek and secure appropriate medical assistance, and effectively carry out medical instructions	Consistently seeks medical advice and assistance when having health concerns. Has the knowledge, skills and resources necessary to effectively carry out medical instructions.	Unable to comply with the details of medical advice, particularly with diet.	Following surgery, Jill must continue to have routine health examinations: compliance must continue. Lifestyle changes will continue to be important after surgery.	• Continue following medical advice and follow-up appointments • Obtain additional sources of information about diet and health	• Reinforce the importance of follow-up care • Continue to be a source of information	• Educate • Support
Be aware of and attend to pathological conditions and side-effects of medical care	Is aware of the links between her condition, lifestyle and diet. Currently there are no obvious physical side-effects. Some psychological difficulties, as restricted foods are often those Jill is particularly fond of.	Is currently unable to manage her pathological condition well at present because of conflicts between personal and professional development and her health concern. Generally manages her condition well, but is not aware of the potential side-effects of surgery at this time.	Surgery will not overcome this conflict. Jill must be aware of an increasing need to manage her diet and weight. Side-effects of surgery can be quite unpleasant. Jill will need education about these.	• Jill can describe and discuss the implications of surgery for her life (e.g. fatigue) and her lifestyle (dietary change)	• Ensure that Jill is aware of some of the side-effects of surgery in general, and of a cholecystectomy in particular • Provide an environment where Jill can discuss some of these issues	• Educate • Support
Modify self-concept to accept need for health care	Willing to accept medical and nursing advice.	Often unable to comply because of conflicts over health and personal/professional development.	Will have to come to terms with the fact that her current lifestyle and ambitions cannot continue unchanged if she is to develop good health.	• Be willing to discuss concerns with members of the health team • Be receptive to information given to her • Verbalise acceptance of self in her current and future situations • Actively seek information • Verbalise understanding of the changes she is likely to encounter following surgery • Acknowledge herself as the individual who has the ultimate responsibility for her own health	• Assess contributing factors to Jill's self-concept, including the following: – knowledge and anxiety levels; – interaction with significant others; – ability to adapt to new situations; – ability to verbalise personal and work conflicts • Ensure accurate information is available to Jill in a form which she can understand • Reinforce explanations given by other members of the health team	• Support • Educate

surgeon and anaesthetist visit and discuss with Jill the nature of the operation, and she signs the consent form.

Jill believes that she will probably not sleep too well during the night, mainly because of the new environment, but does not want anything to help her sleep. She is advised not to take fluids after the evening drinks are passed around. A 'nil by mouth' sign is posted by her bed as a reminder not to allow her anything to eat and drink. This is important to prevent any risk of gastric aspiration during the induction of anaesthesia or during the surgery or recovery period. It is of added importance as in the morning she will be the first patient to have surgery. Her husband arrives during visiting hours and they talk for a while.

Unfortunately, Jill does have a restless night. In the morning, following the taking of routine vital signs, Jill is asked to try to pass urine prior to surgery; this she is able to do. She is also given a pre-medication to help her relax. The theatre nurse arrives at 06.30 to do the pre-operative patient identification and assessment with the primary nurse. This includes ensuring that Jill's name band is correct, that she has been nil-by-mouth for the past few hours, that no make-up is being worn, and that Jill's wedding ring is taped over to avoid the possibility of injury during the operation. Her medical notes are collected as well as the most recent vital-sign recordings. It is noted that Jill has voided urine.

During this time Jill is naturally quite anxious; she answers questions with some hesitation and nervousness. Jill's nurse recognises that this is a stressful time and holds her hand while offering a smile. Jill's husband arrives in time to give her a quick kiss before she is taken to theatre.

Return from surgery

Jill returns from her operation awake, alert and moving all limbs to command. She is in pain, but says that it is not too bad provided she lies still. She complains of being very thirsty and feeling cold. During the operation a cholecystectomy was performed; there were no complications or unexpected occurrences. She has an intravenous line in her left arm and a drain from her right epigastric area. Jill is reminded about these, and asked not to disturb them if at all possible. The nursing staff ensure that there are no kinks or obstructions in any of the tubing, and that the IVI is the prescribed fluid and running at the appropriate rate. There are no signs of inflammation or infiltration around the IV site, and Jill says that the site is not painful.

Her vital signs upon return to the unit are stable and there is no evidence of bleeding around the wound site or into the drain bag. There is a transparent plastic dressing over the wound site which makes observation simple. There are no signs of wound dehiscence. The nursing staff make Jill as comfortable as possible. She is quite anxious and in some pain; it is decided to give her some analgesic medication. Jill is reminded that it is going to be very important to perform deep-breathing and coughing exercises when the pain medication begins to take effect. Soon afterwards the nurse returns with a small pillow which Jill holds against her abdomen while she begins to breathe deeply. This is quite painful for her, but she manages quite well. Jill also acknowledges that the pain medication has greatly eased her discomfort.

Within a couple of hours of arriving back on the unit, and after a warm wash, Jill is feeling more comfortable. She has been able to void urine in a bedpan and has not felt nauseous. Deep-breathing exercises continue; she can now do them unassisted.

EVALUATION

In the first few hours following the return to the unit Jill is quite sleepy and lies still. The nursing staff have to remind Jill to deep-breathe regularly and they encourage her to use the small pillow to hold against herself when she inhales. It is not long before staff observe that Jill no longer needs prompting to deep-breathe and cough as she is now doing this by herself. Instead of directly performing care, staff become supportive of Jill's action and ensure that she has sufficient analgesia to be able to deep-breathe and cough without inordinate pain.

Jill does, however, still need nursing staff to offer direct assistance when trying to manage fluids and foods. While Jill has not been nauseous and has not vomited, no bowel sounds have been heard, and she has not been passing flatus. As a result, she has not been permitted any food yet. Jill is not unduly worried by this and has not been expressing any feelings of hunger. However, it has also meant that she has not been receiving any oral fluids. The IVI which was started during surgery is still being used to manage Jill's fluid requirements. Nursing staff will have to monitor this aspect of Jill's care.

Jill was able to pass urine shortly after returning from theatre and is now asking for a bedpan whenever she needs to void. She has not, however, been able to pass a stool. Again, she is not too worried about this; she is aware that this is common following surgery. Jill also needs considerable assistance with oral hygiene. She is reluctant to move her left arm because of the intravenous line and is concerned that the mouthwash might make her nauseous.

Nursing and physiotherapy staff have been directly helping Jill to swing her legs over the end of the bed to help her get upright. Such exercise is important to prevent one of the complications of bed rest, thrombophlebitis. It is also important for the circulatory system in general, as well as for respiration, and in reducing the risk of Jill developing pressure sores on her sacrum. Jill has been quite reluctant to do this, partly because of the pain involved but also because of her fear that she might pull out her drain or that her stitches might 'burst'. Nursing staff are quick to reassure her that this is unlikely to happen, particularly when there is a nurse or physiotherapist to help her. Despite this reassurance and suitable analgesia given before such activity, it is quite a struggle to get Jill to her feet.

Following such activity, Jill is pleased to return to bed. She lies very still, appearing quite frightened to move. She seems to be resting well, but this is difficult to evaluate. Her eyes are closed, but is she really resting? The ward is busy during the day, with relatively few opportunities for quiet times, so it can be difficult to sleep. Additionally she needs to have her vital signs taken during the day – another disturbance. She cheers up when her husband comes to see her, but is reluctant to engage in conversation with other patients on the ward.

By the end of the first 24 hours post-operatively, Jill is progressively taking on more self-care activities. She is now able to stand by the edge of her bed unassisted and only needs support in walking, for example to the toilet. She has begun to overcome her concerns about the intravenous lines and drainage bag. Consequently she is prepared to become more participative in such activities as brushing her teeth, combing her hair and washing. She has also been greatly reassured by the surgeon and nursing staff reporting that all has gone well, that her vital signs are within expected limits, and that the operation appears not to have had any unexpected side-effects.

Jill's progression has also required that nursing actions be evaluated and modified; the nature of the nursing actions required to help Jill reach her best potential for self-care have changed. By the second day, nursing staff are no longer having to do so many things for her; instead they need only to offer assistance and to support Jill's own efforts. The education role is still important to consider: staff will have to reinforce the advice given to Jill during the time before the operation.

Jill has not spoken much about her future: she is just pleased to be making progress. While nursing staff have included in their interaction with her the need to consider planning her life following discharge, she has made few comments on this subject.

Re-evaluation: day 3

By the third post-operative day, Jill has increased her participation in many aspects of those self-care activities with which nursing staff had previously been helping her. Perhaps the most important improvements from Jill's perspective are that she can now take fluids orally and that the intravenous line has been discontinued. She is particularly pleased about this progress because drinking even small amounts of water has quenched her thirst, and without the intravenous line she has more freedom actually to take care of herself. Her vital signs are unremarkable, and she has opened her bowels for the first time. She is resting much more soundly, and requires much less analgesia. The exception to this move towards a greater independence in self-care is nutrition, which still needs to be managed for her following her operation; she is not taking much solid food as yet.

Many aspects of Jill's care still need resolving. While she is managing much of her own immediate physical care, it has been difficult to assess the extent to which Jill is prepared for her future discharge and for life after returning home. She has been asked several times by nursing staff about her plans for life after the operation, but it is evident that she is taking one day at a time. She has no immediate strategy for altering her lifestyle to incorporate the necessary changes enforced by surgery. Will she continue to drive herself so hard in her professional life? She does not feel able to address these issues at the moment.

Staff continue to offer advice about preparing for discharge, and the dietitian has spent a great deal of time discussing dietary changes which must be undertaken in the future. However, Jill does not seem, as yet, to be able to manage the immediate implications of having to structure her eating habits much more carefully and the effect this may have on her personal and professional life.

Despite this uncertainty, it seems reasonable that Jill will continue her pre-operative compliance with medical advice and see the surgeon and general practitioner as requested. She has already agreed to meet with the dietitian to discuss her future nutritional needs. All this suggests that she is willing to take charge of her health needs. Whether she will make these her top priority remains to be seen.

FOLLOW-UP WORK

Activities

Upon her return home, Jill will have to pay special attention to her diet. She must meet the self-care requisite of maintaining a sufficient intake of appropriate food, in her case a low-fat diet. The following activities can be used to heighten your awareness of the importance of diet in the care of patients, and some of the practical difficulties in obtaining food supplies. You can try them individually or in small groups.

Activity 1

Visit your local supermarket.

- Find out whether there are any brochures or information sheets on food, healthy eating and additives. Examine any information you have found and consider whether it is clear and simple to read and understand.
- Examine the products on the shelves. How are foods labelled? It is clear which are low-fat, low-sugar, or low in cholesterol? Are the ingredients clearly labelled? If in doubt ask the store manager.

If you had to ask for information, how knowledgeable were store staff?

Activity 2

Plan a non-fat diet suitable for Jill. (Remember, Jill can afford to pay more for food than a person living off a pension. Try to be conscious of costs and quality). Perhaps your local library or bookshop may have books on nutrition or diet which would be helpful.

What problems did you encounter planning the low-fat diet? How could these be overcome? Were you able to find any cookery books which cater for special diets?

CHAPTER SIX

Care study: the dependent-care relationship

JONATHON

Jonathon is a talkative and active two-and-a-half-year-old. He lives with his parents, Heather and Norman, and his 15-month-old brother, Bob, in a four-bedroomed house in the Midlands. His mother works three days a week as an occupational therapist at a local hospital, while his father teaches at the local school. The family have a comfortable existence; Jonathon and Bob each have their own bedroom and there is a separate toy room to play in when they cannot go outside. When Heather is at work, both Jonathon and Bob are cared for at a crèche run by the hospital where Heather works. Going to the crèche is the first time that Jonathon and or Bob have been away from their parents, and so far, apart from a few tears when Heather leaves, the boys are enjoying themselves. They have never spent the night away from home without their parents. Unfortunately, their only other relative is Norman's ageing mother, who is unable to travel or to manage the two boys by herself.

Jonathon appears to be developing in a healthy way. He has many teeth, which he enjoys brushing, although he has not as yet visited a dentist. He occasionally sucks his thumb, but only when he is very tired and usually not when he sleeps. He is 90 cm tall and weighs 12.7 kg. He is developing more confidence in his movements, and can walk up and down stairs without falling while holding the banisters. He likes to run everywhere, but still falls quite easily. He is developing greater manual dexterity and improved eye–hand coordination; he is beginning to enjoy ball games much more. His language is developing well: he has an extensive vocabulary and can construct quite complicated sentences. He recognises many different shapes and colours, and has started to recognise consistently letters of the alphabet and numbers.

In general, Jonathon is a healthy child. He has the occasional cold, but apart from contracting rubella at 14 months has experienced no major illness. His parents have ensured that both he and his brother are up to date with their immunisations. Jonathon is an active boy who likes to climb and run. It is following a fall from his climbing frame that Jonathon is admitted to the local hospital, with a suspected fractured leg.

Dependent-care relationships

Jonathon, because of his current stage of development, requires the care of others to meet many of the requisites for a healthy life and normal development. Jonathon is at a point in his life where he is dependent on others to meet many of his self-care needs; the primary dependent-care agent will be his parents, although Orem considers that any responsible adult can meet the dependent-care needs of another person. The other major source of care will be provided by nursing staff in the form of nursing agency. It is anticipated that there will be many aspects of Jonathon's care that will require direct care from nursing staff, assisted by his parents. This puts Jonathon into a complicated combination of roles, because there will be times when he will be a 'patient' and others when he will be a 'child'. The roles of Heather and Norman may also vacillate, between 'parent' and direct 'care-givers'; in both roles they will be fulfilling some dependent-care agency.

It will also be important to understand the nature of the dependent-care systems that Heather and Norman have adopted with Jonathon – how they normally look after him, their daily care routines, and (for example) their use of special words. Specifically, Orem (1991, p.108) suggests that the following information be obtained to assist in the assessment process:

1 establish what Jonathon and his dependent-care agents (parents) customarily do in terms of their caring to meet universal self-care requisites, and the frequency of these practices;
2 establish what developmental self-care requisites are understood, and the care measures used to meet them;
3 know about any obstacles that may interfere with the regularly-used caring methods adopted to meet universal and developmental self-care requisites;
4 establish the presence or absence of health practices to meet health-deviation self-care requisites;

5 establish how adopting a dependent-care system articulates with normal patterns of daily living.

Jonathon's mother will be an important provider of this care, along with nursing staff. In this situation both Heather and the nursing staff will be dependent-care agents – that is, the people taking action on Jonathon's behalf – however, Heather is likely to take the role of *primary* dependent-care agent: it is she who has been meeting most of Jonathon's care needs since his birth. The arrangement whereby she and Bob can stay with Jonathon in hospital permits her to continue her caring role. This is an essential feature of the care plan; this togetherness will help provide the appropriate environment for care to be given. It will be important to Jonathon in his struggle to understand what is happening to him, and will provide him with comfort and reassurance. At the same time it will permit Heather to retain her self-confidence and self-esteem about her mothering abilities. It should therefore minimise anxiety both for Jonathon and and for his mother.

Dependent-care limitations

Some care limitations are obvious. Heather does not know a great deal about the physical care of her son now that he is in hospital. She will also have to consider the care of Bob and herself. Although Norman can come along first thing in the mornings and in the evenings, there are long periods of time that she must spend (and is willing to spend) with Jonathon. She must rely on the hospital timetables for the provision of food. There are also technical aspects of care which will need to be performed by trained nursing staff, so she will have to share the care of her son.

Heather has concerns about her ability to look after Jonathon. She knows she can comfort him in times of hurt and when he is tired, but what will happen if he experiences great pain or discomfort? What of the boredom? How will she structure the day to keep an active boy entertained throughout it? How will she adapt to this alteration in her routine; can she manage?

It is possible to devise a plan of care which involves both Jonathon and his mother. While there are many physical aspects of Jonathon's care which it is very important to consider, managing the anxiety, fear and distress of both mother and son regarding hospitalisation must be given prominence in the care plan.

ASSESSMENT

Jonathon and his mother are brought to the children's ward of the local hospital after being seen in the accident and emergency department. Following a series of X-rays, the extent of his injuries has been determined: he has a fractured right femur. This will require traction, and a stay in hospital.

Most of the information required to assess Jonathon is obtained from his mother. Jonathon is obviously in pain and is clinging on to his mother's hand. As long as she is close by, though, he has been cooperative with the care given so far. Taking X-rays was problematic as Heather could not always be as close to Jonathon as he would have liked. Clearly Jonathon is under some stress during the assessment but he says nothing throughout the whole process. He stays close to his mother and hugs his teddy bear.

Orem recognises that there are going to be situations when the primary provider of care is not the person – adult or child – himself, but another, perhaps a parent. This is the nature of the relationship between Jonathon and his mother. Orem (1991, p.242) details that in the care of children, nursing staff must select ways of assisting patients that are consistent with their age and stage of growth and development; specifically, caring for, acting or doing things for the child and providing the child with an environment consistent with supporting and promoting development and essential nursing considerations. It must also be recognised that children may want to learn aspects of their own care: this too must be part of the therapeutic and developmental environment which is cultivated.

However, the relationship of a young child with his parent or parents is important when the child is hospitalised. While the assessment details must concentrate on the child, Jonathon's mother also must be considered. For the purpose of this assessment and care plan, the actions and concerns of parent and child cannot be considered in isolation.

Following negotiations with hospital staff, it is arranged for Heather to stay with Jonathon on a 24-hour basis. Bob can also stay, if necessary.

Universal self-care requisites

The maintenance of a sufficient intake of air

Jonathon is able to breathe normally through his nose and mouth.

No wheezing can be heard. Recently he has had a head cold and he has a running nose. He hates having others wipe his nose, and if given a handkerchief he will do it himself. He has no cough. Heather tells the nurse that he does not usually have any breathing difficulties but does snore loudly at night.

The maintenance of a sufficient intake of water

Heather is asked about what Jonathon eats, and from this it emerges that he will eat and drink most things given to him. He drinks plenty of milk and particularly likes apple juice. He usually drinks from a glass, which he can manage without spilling; he sometimes likes to use a straw. He generally drinks several glasses of fluids each day. He likes to have a drink of water just before going to bed, and he has a drink by his bedside which he may have if he wakes during the night.

The maintenance of a sufficient intake of food

When eating, Jonathon still reverts at times to using his hands, although he is beginning to use a knife and fork. Fortunately he does try to eat most things, particularly liking sausages. He is beginning to learn some of the social skills surrounding eating, such as not bringing toys to the table, and washing his hands before starting to eat.

The provision of care associated with the elimination processes and excrements

Jonathon is only partially toilet-trained. For the most part he is still in nappies. During the day if he is put on the toilet he will pass urine, Jonathon's word for urine being 'pee pee'. He still has accidents during the day, and requires nappies through the night, but there are some mornings when he wakes up dry. When attending the crèche, he often wears pants. This makes him feel more grown up, and with plenty of supervision he rarely wets himself. At this time, Jonathon has not developed any obvious routine with his bowels. Only on rare occasions is he able to pass a stool in the toilet, and for the most part requires Heather or Norman to clean him.

The maintenance of a balance between activity and rest

Both Jonathon's parents acknowledge that he is a very active boy, rushing around and sometimes being careless. He frequently falls when running and has many bruises on his arms and legs from such falls. He particularly likes a toy car on which he can sit and race around the garden, a pastime which often leads to him falling off and hurting himself. He likes to use the climbing frame, the slide and the swing in the back garden. He is becoming more adventurous on this equipment. He also likes to play indoors, making buildings out of construction blocks and making 'music' on his toy piano. He can recognise many shapes, animals, numbers and objects. He often wants his mother or father to read to him. This, coupled with judicious viewing of children's educational television, seems to have made Jonathon enjoy books.

The result of all this activity is that Jonathon does become quite tired in the afternoons and needs to rest. There are structured rest times at the crèche he attends, and on days when he is at home he often needs to go to sleep during the day. This can sometimes be a stressful time for both Jonathon and his mother. When Jonathon gets tired it becomes progressively more difficult to reason with him, and often he has to be carried to bed crying. However, he soon settles and after about an hour and a half wakes up refreshed. At bedtime either Heather or Norman reads him and his brother a story, which they really enjoy. Generally he sleeps soundly through the night. He has a favourite teddy bear which he sleeps with. He wakes, almost like clockwork, at about seven o'clock in the morning.

The maintenance of a balance between solitude and social integration

Jonathon is a friendly and affectionate boy, smiling and laughing as he plays. Before starting at the crèche, there had been few opportunities to play with children of his own age. He does play with his brother, but only for short periods. He does, however, share toys with Bob and even tries to comfort him when he is hurt. Since starting the crèche, however, Jonathon has had the opportunity to mix with many children, particularly older ones; he has even started to understand the concept of 'boys' and 'girls'. In mixing with older children Jonathon seems to have overcome any shyness or reluctance to participate in games or playing: he has become much more outgoing and adventurous.

91

The preventions of hazards to life, human functioning, and human well-being

Jonathon is at an age of great risk of physical injury. While he is careful in many aspects of play, he is still careless in others. He does not yet have sufficient judgement, for example, to know when to slow down on his car; the result is usually a fall. His parents have been very firm with him about the ideas of 'hot' and 'cold', particularly in the kitchen and when water taps are involved; he can associate 'red' with 'hot'. He has learned the importance of staying close by his parents when they go out in the car or when walking by roads. Obviously, however, he requires his parents to manage many aspects of home safety for him and to provide the essential elements of a balanced diet and secure family environment.

Normacy

The centre of Jonathon's life must be that of being part of a family. He obviously gains the necessary love, security and encouragement from his parents. He is encouraged to be inquisitive and ask questions, and to explore and find out – whenever possible by himself. He likes affection and being hugged by his parents, who in return gain great pleasure from playing with him and Bob. He likes to be with them. Heather and Norman both feel a little guilt about sending Jonathon and Bob to the crèche while they work; however, they try to ensure that both boys are given as much attention and affection as possible during the times when they can be together.

Developmental self-care requisites

Erikson (1963) introduced a cultural and societal perspective to the development of humans throughout their life span, and introduced the idea of the 'eight ages of man'. Viewing Jonathon in Erikson's terms, the child between the ages of 18 months and three years is facing a crisis over the need for autonomy versus shame and doubt. Jonathon at this age has begun to realise that he has the ability to make his own judgements and a sense of self. Jonathon asserts his own will, trying to achieve autonomy or self-determination. There is a conflict here, however, as Jonathon also realises there are some limitations to his autonomy: he is still heavily dependent on his parents for support in almost all he does. Jonathon must somehow strike a balance between what he is obviously able to do, what he feels it is safe to do, and those activities which he is not as yet ready to do. For example, Jonathon can begin to undress himself, but is not sure whether it is 'safe' to hug all the nursing staff.

The so-called 'terrible twos', which Jonathon at times demonstrates, is a natural manifestation of the need for autonomy to emerge. Jonathon is changing from a highly dependent infant towards a child capable of making some decisions for himself. He is no longer content to accept the decisions of others unquestioningly; he wants to assert his own opinions, beliefs and wishes. The result with Jonathon is commonly a loud 'No!' Jonathon frequently exhibits this 'negativism'. Heather and Norman work hard with Jonathon to lessen the frequency of these outbursts, but it is not always easy to find a suitable level of control which permits Jonathon self-expression while maintaining a safe environment and some sort of order at home.

Health-deviation self-care requisites

Heather, in the course of her professional experience, has seen many people who have experienced similar injuries. Despite this exposure, she is quite upset and anxious about Jonathon's situation. She puts on a brave face in an attempt to avoid letting Jonathon know she is worried.

Following Jonathon's fall, she took swift action and called the emergency services. Despite her clinical background she is not well versed in the care and management of her son's fracture; she is worried about whether he will walk 'normally' again. Heather and Jonathon appear genuinely willing to follow whatever advice or instructions are offered to them, and provided they can stay together, Jonathon seems to be more settled. Heather knows that some of the procedures that Jonathon must have performed are going to be painful, but she is unsure how best to communicate this to him. She is not sure how to deal with him should he start screaming with pain or crying that he wants to go home. Heather appears to realise that Jonathon does need medical intervention and that hospital, for the time being, is the appropriate place to be, but she is unsure how she will react to Jonathon's situation. There are also many other worries. Who will look after Bob when Norman is at work? Heather is unsure of her ability to look after Jonathon; this is having an adverse affect on her self-esteem and her feelings of competence as a mother.

PLANNING

System of care

The need to have a plan of care is discussed with Heather, as is the need to distribute the responsibilities for Jonathon's care. Heather is very keen to be involved in as many aspects of Jonathon's care as possible, as is his father. Further discussions ensure that Heather does not feel she is being pressured or coerced into participating in her son's care. Reassurance is thereby given that her mothering role is very important to Jonathon, but when she feels particularly anxious, unsure or simply exhausted, she can turn to nursing staff for support and assistance. The care required by Jonathon is likely to invoke the full range of nursing systems suggested by Orem – supportive/educative, and partly and wholly compensatory systems of care. Specifically, caring for, acting or doing for, and providing an environment which supports and promotes both Jonathon's and his mother's self-care abilities, will need to be developed.

Objectives of the care plan

There are two principal components of the nursing care of Jonathon and his mother to be considered, involving short-term and long-term objectives. The focus of this care plan will not be on the technical aspects of the care of Jonathon's fractures (wholly compensatory), but on the psychosocial and developmental aspects of nursing interventions. The needs of Jonathon and his mother must be prioritised, as is reflected in the following objectives.

In the shorter term (the first week of hospitalisation), the following are going to be important.

1 ensuring that Heather and Jonathon can be together as much as possible; in particular, to provide a facility where she can stay with him overnight if necessary (supportive/educative and partial-compensatory);

2 ensuring that Jonathon and Heather have knowledge about their situation appropriate for their developmental level (supportive/ educative);

3 reducing anxiety for Heather and Jonathon (supportive/educative and partial-compensatory);

4 reducing fear in Jonathon and his mother (supportive/educative and partial-compensatory).

Longer-term nursing care aims must be to provide an appropriate environment for Jonathon and his mother to develop in a normal way. Given that this hospitalisation is going to be a major crisis in their lives, it is imperative that any potential physical or psychosocial problems be resolved without lasting effects.

INTERVENTION

The short-term objectives given above form the basis of the care plan for Jonathon and his mother. It is assumed that Heather will be acting as a dependent-care agent. Emerging from the nursing assessment of Jonathon and his parents, the following key aspects of dependent care can be identified: knowledge deficit, fear and anxiety, and family coping. Each of these three aspects of care will require the development of desired care outcomes for Jonathon, and negotiation between Heather (in her role as dependent-care agent) and the nursing staff.

Knowledge deficit

Heather has a knowledge deficit about Jonathon's condition. If she is to be able to manage his care to the high standards she expects of herself, learning must take place. Specifically, nursing staff must determine when Heather and Jonathon are ready to learn about daily care. This may involve Heather finding new ways of managing many of Jonathon's universal self-care requisites, such as elimination. Specific attention must be given to the developmental differences between Jonathon and his mother; these will influence the methods of teaching to take place. Heather, in particular, must be motivated to learn. Fortunately this does not seem to be a problem, as she has shown every indication of wanting to learn. Involving Heather and Jonathon in the learning process will be important. Allowing Heather to determine her own priorities for learning, and weighing these against the nursing staff's perceptions of priorities, will establish the basis for a negotiated learning plan. Appropriate learning objectives and teaching methods must be employed, based upon developmental level and readiness to learn. Environmental factors are also important. Naturally, times when Heather is tired may not be the best to begin education sessions.

It is also important to educate Jonathon about what has happened to him and why some of the procedures performed on him must be done. This interaction must be pitched at a developmental level appropriate for him. This is important because Jonathon is at an age which Piaget (1952) considers to be 'pre-operational'. Olds and Papalia (1986), in reviewing Piaget's work, suggest that this means, amongst other things, that Jonathon may interpret some unpleasant or painful experiences as being 'punishment'. Care must be taken in what is said to him as well as the way in which care is given. In addressing some of these issues, play and acting out some of the things that will happen to Jonathon throughout the day can be a very important aspect of his care. Dressing up his favourite toys with bandages similar to Jonathon's might be one simple technique to use. Additionally, Heather, nursing staff and the play therapist have an important role in correcting any misconceptions that Jonathon may express about his care, and in reminding him that he is not being punished.

Desired outcomes

Jonathon will:

- express in his own way, either verbally or through play, what has happened to him physically, and why he is in hospital (away from home);
- express in his own way, either verbally or through play, what he understands about the care being given to him: this might involve him role-playing with his teddy bear;
- indicate that he recognises that he has not been a naughty boy, and that being in hospital is not a punishment for anything he may have done: he might state factually that he fell from his climbing frame.

Heather will:

- actively participate in the learning process by showing interest in Jonathon's care (through the use of verbal or non-verbal expression);
- exhibit greater confidence in her abilities to look after Jonathon, and take increased responsibility for learning (this might be demonstrated by asking questions or seeking information from other sources, such as books and magazines);
- demonstrate or explain progressively more understanding of Jonathon's condition, and in appropriate situations perform care for Jonathon, giving reasons for her actions;

- begin to show signs of making lifestyle changes as a result of her son's injury during the time he is hospitalised: this might be demonstrated by her being able to re-order life priorities.

Fear and anxiety

It will be important for nursing staff to assess and monitor both Jonathon's and his mother's anxiety levels. Nursing staff must be sensitive to the verbal and non-verbal responses that Heather might be giving. She may use denial, or have a short attention span. Another gauge of levels of anxiety could be the family dynamics when Norman and Bob are present. This may give some indication of the family's coping methods. Perhaps the most important role for nursing staff will be simply making time to be available to listen and talk. It is important for Heather to have the opportunity to ask questions in a calm environment where she feels comfortable expressing her fears and anxieties and where she does not feel threatened or uneasy about expressing her emotions, such as sadness or anger. Nursing staff must be able to discuss issues of fear openly with Heather and Jonathon, and they must be comfortable replying. There is therefore the need for a trusting relationship between Heather, Jonathon and nursing staff. There will be times when Jonathon and Heather will be frightened: nursing staff will have to help Heather and Jonathon identify their feelings of fear or anxiety and suggest ways of dealing with them. This is important because an increased anxiety level may influence Heather's ability to learn about Jonathon's condition and to manage specific aspects of care.

There should also be some planning for times of anxiety and fear. Some procedures are likely to cause Jonathon discomfort and he will cry. This may cause Heather to become anxious and fearful. Sometimes fear can be the result of possessing insufficient information: an important nursing role will be to give appropriate information to Heather and Jonathon regarding developments in his condition; secrecy or half-truths can destroy a therapeutic relationship. Preparing them in advance of procedures may lessen the impact of nursing actions. At all times, however, nursing staff should be aware of a subtle balance between how much information and preparation the nursing staff think is important and how much Heather or Jonathon can actually manage.

Desired outcomes

Jonathon will demonstrate the following behaviours. He will:

- accept comfort from nursing and other hospital staff (such as the doctor or the play therapist) as well as from his mother;
- react calmly to nursing or care procedures carried out either by nursing staff or by his mother;
- tolerate being separated from his mother for short periods, without crying for her;
- begin to participate in play activities on the children's unit.

Heather will demonstrate the following behaviours. She will:

- feel comfortable expressing her fears to nursing staff;
- demonstrate, either verbally or non-verbally, ways of dealing with her fears;
- seek alternative ways of reducing fear and anxiety, for example discussing concerns with medical or nursing staff and talking to other parents on the unit.

Family coping

The impact that Jonathon's hospitalisation is having on his parents' lives is likely to be considerable. It will be important for the family to be able to adapt to the changes forced upon them. Nursing staff will have a role to play in helping them to adapt to such changes. Wherever possible it will be important to evaluate the family as a unit. Particularly important will be the need to assess further the family's hopes and fears, and their plans to deal with their life changes. These will indicate the communication pattern of the family.

This pattern is important when helping the family 'grow' as a result of Jonathon's experience. Nursing staff can provide a role model for Heather and Norman, as well as helping to promote open communication and problem-solving. Nursing staff may also be able to support parents so that they can meet their needs or learn new ways of dealing with their concerns. It might also be useful for nursing staff to introduce them to other parents who are experiencing similar worries and concerns; this might offer reassurance.

Desired outcomes

Jonathon will demonstrate the following behaviours. He will:

- accept comfort from either his mother or father;
- sleep well;
- join in play activities with his brother when possible.

Heather and Norman will:

- show some evidence of evaluating their lives and being prepared to make changes;
- express feelings of confidence and satisfaction with the care they are giving to their son;
- express feelings that their relationship is growing as a result of this life-event.

EVALUATION

While most of Jonathon's care proceeded without major problems, some problems occurred that required sensitive management and demonstrated the complex nature of caring for children. Essentially, Jonathon's coming into hospital is a health-deviation self-care requisite, at a time in his life when he has special developmental self-care needs and is in a dependent-care relationship with his mother and nursing staff.

This complex situation was highlighted when Jonathon started to have sleepless nights. It was difficult to help him settle, as the environment was unusual; he did not have familiar objects surrounding him. There were strange noises and lights in the unit which he was unfamiliar with. There were also times when his parents needed to go home – to check on the house, to receive mail, to shower, and so on. Sometimes Jonathon would wake up startled and disorientated, looking for his mother; he cried if she was not in sight. Nursing staff tried to explain to him in language appropriate to his developmental level that she would be back soon and that she had not left him for long. He would cry and the nursing staff would find it hard to console him; it was difficult to communicate the concept of time to a tired child.

It did not take long for Heather to become familiar with the basic care of Jonathon while in hospital; she can now perform competently many activities she previously could not. She has demonstrated an increased knowledge about the more technical aspects of Jonathon's care, helping nursing staff with their duties, bringing to their attention changes in Jonathon's condition, and asking more appropriate and detailed questions.

The same can be said for Jonathon himself. He now freely verbalises that he is in hospital because 'leg hurts' and appears to understand that nursing staff must perform some aspects of his care that his mother cannot. He is happy for nursing staff to help him, and no longer fights or cries when they appoach, as he did when he was first admitted to the unit. He also shows people his teddy bear which has a bandage in place on its leg, and says 'teddy broke leg as well'. Generally, his mother is content with the information and knowledge she now possesses; certainly she is now confident to participate actively in his care.

While there are times when Jonathon and his mother can play and for a while put out of their minds the fact that they are in hospital together, there are others when Jonathon does become anxious and frightened. This usually occurs when the medical staff come round. Unfortunately Jonathon has associated the white-coated medical staff with pain and unpleasant experiences. When the doctor comes to see how his patient is progressing, Jonathon ceases being a happy and smiling child; instead he stops speaking and clings to his mother and his teddy. On one occasion when the medical staff visited and Heather was not there, Jonathon started crying loudly and shouting for his mother. Happily, nursing staff were able to comfort him, but the incident was unfortunate as Jonathon's doctor is a kind and gentle person.

Heather, when discussing Jonathon's care with the nurse in charge of the unit, expresses her feelings that for the most part she is much less anxious and frightened about her son's condition. She has overcome her initial concerns of 'will he live?' and is now concerned with how best to make his time in hospital as settled as possible. She tries hard to help him understand what is going on, and this seems to be working.

While Jonathon is responding well to the care plan devised for him, the stress of the change in family living arrangements is causing a great strain on the family as a whole. After only a few days of sleeping in the hospital with Jonathon, and sometimes Bob, Heather is looking very tired and exhausted. She feels it is her responsibility to be with Jonathon all the time. This has put added responsibilities on Norman, who already has a very busy day. Sometimes Heather and Norman are seen to be arguing about how best to manage the family affairs. The family does not seem to be coping well at this time. Norman has suggested that Jonathon is now settled in the unit sufficiently well for Heather to come home, catch up on sleep and relax for a night. Heather is unable, as yet, to do this. The nursing staff are aware of this situation, which seems to be quite common when parents stay with their children on a 24-hour basis, and intend to encourage her to go home for a while.

Jonathon's physical condition is improving well. He is increasingly less anxious and frightened by his new environment, and has said that he likes the play therapist when she visits him. His mother, as dependent-care agent, is also managing his care well. She has become increasingly knowledgeable and her own level of anxiety has decreased. New problems have occurred, as Heather is not taking good care of herself. This must become the new focus of nursing intervention.

FOLLOW-UP WORK

Questions

The following questions can also be used as group exercises. As with other care plans, small groups of 6–8 people could address the issues which follow; 20–30 minutes' discussion on each should be sufficient. Remember to nominate a note-taker. Use your lecturer or facilitator to help your discussions: he or she may be particularly helpful if you feel that you cannot make any progress with an issue or are at an impasse.

1 From the information given in this care plan, to what extent do you agree with the priorities of care adopted? What alternative aspects of care would you want to have seen included? List and discuss your own priorities for Jonathon's and his mother's care.
2 Identify and discuss alternative strategies for the management of knowledge, anxiety and fear in Jonathon and his mother. How successful were the approaches adopted in this care study?
3 What are the possible consequences of hospitalisation on Jonathon? Do you think that the care plan minimises these?
4 Discuss the importance of role-play for children who are hospitalised. Apart from those described in the care plan, what other types of role-play could you adopt with Jonathon?
5 What are the major problems in planning patient care when a dependent-care relationship already exists, as with Jonathon and

his mother? How could you plan to meet both their needs? What of Bob – is there a nursing responsibility for him as well?

6 If Heather had not wanted to participate in Jonathon's care, how would this have influenced the care plan? What do you consider the main aims of care in this situation? What would your own new priorities be?

7 Given that many approaches to the care of children are influenced by the child's developmental level, how would you determine the extent of Jonathon's knowledge of his situation? Is this an important consideration in planning his care? If so, why?

8 How useful and important are the perspectives of Erikson and Piaget in the process of assessing, planning and evaluating care? Do such theorists have an important role to play?

9 Should nursing staff encourage patients or other care-givers to be involved in continuing to provide care in hospital, as they have been doing in their home environment? If you do believe this to be a nursing role, what strategies might you adopt to encourage people to participate?

10 Heather clearly felt that it was her responsibility to stay with Jonathon during his hospitalisation. What approaches could be used to discuss with Heather her going home for periods in the day? What if she insisted on staying?

11 Clearly there has been increasing stress and tension between Heather and Norman; Jonathon's hospitalisation has brought about enforced changes in their lives. Is it a nursing responsibility to become involved in such problems? If so, what approaches might you adopt to help them?

Activities

The following activities can be carried out individually or in small groups.

Activity 1

Prior to coming into hospital, Jonathon and his mother probably had ideas or expectations about being a patient. The following activities are designed to examine these images.

Visit your local bookshop and toy shop and see whether you can find any materials about children going into hospital. If you find books, what images and descriptions do they have in common? For example:

- How is hospital life for a child portrayed?
- What role do parents have in the literature?
- How are nursing, medical and other professional staff portrayed?
- How do the media convey their image of nursing and health care? Is it an accurate one?

Activity 2

An important aspect of Jonathon's care is to reduce anxiety by informing Jonathon and his mother about life in hospital. Bearing in mind Jonathon's age and developmental level, create a story or game to tell Jonathon about hospital life. Consider the following:

- How would you involve his parents in your story or game?
- How will his teddy feature in the story or game?
- What will you say about nursing staff and their care?
- How could your activity differ if Jonathon were bored or anxious?

CHAPTER SEVEN

Care study: community psychiatric care

VICTORIA

Born in the early 1920s in a small fishing village on the south coast of England, Victoria had a strict upbringing. She was given little opportunity to see or explore different places or take many decisions for herself. This was largely due to her father, a rigid and inflexible man who ruled his wife and three children in an environment of firm discipline. He physically disciplined the children even when they were in their early twenties. He demanded respect from his family but instead they were somewhat frightened of him.

Victoria's mother Dorothy was a hard-working woman who looked after the children and kept a boarding house for visitors to the town. Dorothy had considerable experience of hardship and personal loss; three brothers were drowned in World War I and she lost a child around the same time. In Victoria's childhood money was short, and there were few luxuries. Outings were very rare, with the exception of an annual visit to the hop fields of Kent; many families from the town would travel there together by bus and pick hops for some extra money. Here the children had the opportunity to run and play, free from the usual constraints of home.

Victoria was the middle child, and by all accounts was quiet, placid and easy-going. She liked to help in the house, particularly when visitors came to stay. She had friends, most of whom lived in the streets nearby, but was never particularly adventurous at play. She preferred to keep close to her parents and rarely explored new surroundings. Her sister Gladys, four years older, had her own friends and did not play much with her. Her brother Joe was six years younger, and Victoria was often left to look after him when she would rather have been doing other things.

Victoria enjoyed going to school but left at fourteen as was customary at the time. She realises with hindsight that she actually received almost no education at all. Victoria sees her school times as happy ones but wishes that her writing and numerical abilities were better. She has felt embarrassed and hindered by the fact that she has difficulty spelling and writing reasonable English.

The outbreak of World War II heralded a great change in Victoria's and her family's lives. The town, because of its strategic position, was frequently the target of bombings. Victoria's father became important with the home defence and fire service and was away from home a great deal; her mother lived life as best she could under wartime threat. Most of the young children in the town were evacuated to Devon. Gladys moved to the munitions factory, Joe became a paratrooper and Victoria joined the Auxiliary Territorial Service and was sent to a training establishment to serve in the officers' mess.

This posting was the first major move from home. Victoria recalls with fond memories making new friends, and meeting men for the first time. She liked the service work, which reminded her of the days when she looked after visitors to her mother's boarding house. She thinks she gave good and courteous service – something to be proud of, she says.

After the war, Victoria left the services and went to work in the restaurant of a local department store. It was work she was familiar with and enjoyed doing. It was about this time that Victoria met Michael. He had spent many years at sea, had seen much of the world and a great deal of life. He had been imprisoned for some years during the war and this had made him very resourceful and quite self-centred at times. They were married in the town a few months after meeting.

Michael got on well with Victoria's parents. He particularly liked her father, in whom he admired straight no-nonsense talking. Victoria and Michael were able to gather sufficient funds to rent a small house close to Victoria's parents; Michael had work in a small television shop and their lives were quite stable. Then Michael was offered a much better job in another part of the country. After a brief discussion, he decided to take it, and they left Victoria's home town.

This move, while good for Michael, was very traumatic for Victoria. The small village they moved to had only two small shops; the next nearest town was six miles away. They had a car, but Michael needed this for work; Victoria was not able to drive and felt she could not learn. They were about a hundred miles from

Victoria's home, but would visit occasionally at the weekends and at Christmas. Victoria was not very happy where she was living. Being away from family, friends and a familiar environment was painful for her.

After about two years, Victoria became pregnant. During her pregnancy, Victoria spent a great deal of time at her parents', as Michael was working long hours and often came home very late. He would, however, visit her most weekends. She gave birth to a son, James, who became the focus of their lives. Victoria now had something to keep her busy. Family life began to take on a routine. Michael made the decisions for the family; he earned all the family's income and felt *he* could decide how it was spent. In all financial matters, Victoria was kept ignorant; she never had a cheque book or even went into a bank. She was given her 'house money' with which she had to feed and clothe the family. Saturday was their weekly shopping outing. She rarely went out at any other time; with poor transportation, it was almost impossible to go anywhere to meet new people. Although they were not like the people she had grown up with, she did begin to make friends with some neighbours, and, in time began to feel more at home in the community. Michael, however, remained set in his ways and Victoria was never given the opportunity to become more involved in the running of the household.

James grew up without any major problems, although quite differently from his parents. Neither of them had any education beyond the age of fourteen, yet James went to university and gained a degree in engineering. This opened doors overseas, and he went to South Africa to work. Victoria hated James being away. She had become used to him being at university and coming home regularly. Now she saw him only once a year, usually at Christmas.

James had been overseas for some years when Michael died suddenly after a heart attack. Michael and Victoria had been married for thirty-five years, and the impact of his death was devastating. Victoria had few people to turn to. By now her parents and her brother had died and her sister, who was not in good health and could not drive, was not able to do much to help. James came home for the funeral and was faced with the daunting task of trying to prepare his mother to manage many self-care activities where hitherto Michael had always provided for her. He helped her sell their house and move back to her home town, near her sister. Shortly after this, he moved back to England close to where his mother lived. However, this did not help the increasing feelings of anxiety that Victoria was experiencing about her ability to cope with life.

Current situation

It is against this background that Victoria's anxiety problems have developed. She experiences physical manifestations such as tachycardia, sweating, flushes and vertigo when faced with new or unfamiliar situations. Her anxieties are preventing her from living a full and productive life. She feels unable to travel by herself to visit friends or relatives, yet she is happy to walk and take local buses in the familiar environment of her home town. What is particularly painful for her is that she cannot take a bus to visit her son and young grandchildren, even though it is a direct route. Day-to-day changes in routine are increasingly difficult to deal with. Even receiving letters is at times anxiety-provoking: a letter may require her to make a decision. Victoria realises that she should be able to enjoy life. She is seventy years of age but does not feel old, and she is generally in good health. She has had elevated blood pressure for a number of years but this has been well controlled by medication. She has no financial worries, as Michael ensured she could own her own house and had invested money to supplement her old-age pension. She wants for nothing materially.

This situation has been going on for about eighteen months, but recently her son, realising that his mother's anxiety is preventing her from enjoying a full life, spoke about it to his mother's general practitioner. The GP was receptive to Victoria's needs and has asked Susan, the community psychiatric nurse attached to the surgery, to visit her. James who has a good relationship with his mother, has been talking to Victoria for some time about her difficulties. At first she was reluctant to see or to talk to anybody about her situation. It has only been recently, when her eldest grandson became old enough to ask her to visit, that she has realised something must be done. If it can be done in her own home, so much the better.

ASSESSMENT

An Orem framework is used as a foundation for assessing and planning Victoria's care. Upon Susan's first visit, James is present with his mother. Victoria is tense and unsure of what to say, but after a short period she feels confident enough to speak to Susan alone with James in another room. It is apparent that Victoria has no obvious physical difficulties (she has been examined recently by her doctor); she is eating well and does not have any difficulties getting to sleep at night. The house is well maintained and clean.

Susan talks to Victoria about her life history and begins to examine more closely the nature of her difficulties. In particular, Susan asks Victoria what she thinks is causing the anxiety. Victoria, somewhat hesitantly, blames her problems on a poor education, harsh upringing, moving away from her home town, and Michael's death. It is apparent from Victoria's conversation that she misses Michael a great deal, and even with James living close by, she is greatly upset. Family and friends initially rallied around to help, but her closest companions are themselves older now. They cannot travel easily to see Victoria, and she sometimes has difficulty meeting them. 'I've never had to do much for myself, now I have to do everything. I just can't manage so much as I used to, these days', she says.

Victoria goes on to explain that she can often feel an 'attack', as she calls it, coming on. 'I feel as if noises get louder and colours brighter, and my head begins to spin. My heart starts to pound and I have to get away.' It is at this point that Victoria usually feels like fainting, though she cannot remember ever actually doing so. These events happen unexpectedly when she faces a new or different situation, or at any time when Victoria is made the centre of public observation, as when being asked a question in a shop. Her response is almost always to leave the situation. Relatively soon after this she feels much better and can resume her daily routines.

It emerges from these conversations that Victoria is having difficulty in meeting all her universal self-care requisites. While she appears to have no problem meeting physical universal self-care requisites, both maintaining a balance between solitude and social interaction and the promotion of normacy are difficult.

Dealing with developmental self-care requisites raises some difficult issues for Susan. Victoria has experienced considerable emotional turmoil and a number of key life-events. The death of her husband is an obvious recent one. Much more difficult to assess is the impact of events which occurred many years ago. How significant is the knowledge of Victoria's change in living conditions when she moved from her home town, or the relative educational deprivation she experienced as a child? How can this information be used?

Health-deviation self-care requisites also pose some concerns for Susan as she develops a therapeutic relationship with Victoria. On past history, Victoria has been compliant with medical advice and intervention. However, her self-concept and self-image are poor, as is her self-confidence. These are key health-deviation self-care deficits which need to be addressed.

In summary, Victoria does have some self-care limitations. These are confined mostly to non-physical self-care requisites. In particular, she has difficulty meeting the universal self-care requisites of maintaining a balance between solitude and social interaction and of promoting normacy. There are also developmental requisites to take into account. The death of her husband is a major life-event and must be considered carefully with any intervention. Victoria has experienced a series of life-events which, according to Orem, can have a major impact upon the development of an individual. These include a harsh upbringing and possible educational deprivation. These factors must be considered when planning care. Finally, Victoria has a poor self-image which might be considered a health-deviation self-care limitation. Why image problems have occurred is often difficult to determine, but Victoria has accepted a series of jobs which placed her in 'service' roles, such as in the ATS and in the restaurant. This attitude may have been compounded by the nature of her relationship with Michael, in which he made the decisions and she simply accepted them. There appear to have been few opportunities for Victoria to learn or develop essential self-care skills in decision-making, communication and socialisation.

PLANNING

Based on Susan's assessment, several approaches are adopted for Victoria's care. This involves the use of Susan's own therapeutic skills, such as touch and soft voice. Additionally, Susan decides to include time to explore with Victoria the nature of her anxieties, and to examine in particular the impact of her husband's death. Finally, there will be some behavioural exercises; for example, Susan will accompany Victoria to places or events which have the potential to be anxiety-provoking. Victoria has agreed to participate in this range of therapeutic interventions, something Susan believes it is very important to have achieved before attempting any lifestyle or behavioural changes. The way in which the interventions are to be used is discussed at length between the two of them.

Initially, they will continue to develop their confidence in each other. Susan will examine the nature of Victoria's feelings towards her dead husband to establish the nature of her grief and her expression of it. Additionally, several simple mental and physical techniques will be introduced to help Victoria become more aware of the events preceding an anxiety attack, and to help her manage anxiety when it occurs. These discussions will take place prior to any behavioural interventions.

In terms of a nursing system for intervention, both Victoria and Susan agree that a supportive/educative stance would be the most appropriate starting point for their interactions. Susan will explain to Victoria more about the nature of anxiety and help develop methods to improve the management of her fears. This will be done in a supportive and understanding environment. When it comes to going into the community, Susan acknowledges that the nature of her nursing intervention may change from supportive/educative to a partly compensatory one, to assist Victoria to manage everyday events. Finally, should a situation occur in which Victoria does experience high levels of anxiety which she appears not to be able to manage, Susan is prepared to adopt a wholly compensatory role, and actually to remove Victoria from the anxiety-provoking environment. This approach to planning care is different from that normally expected when using Orem, in that wholly or partly compensatory nursing systems are usually adopted first. Then, as the individual makes improvement, these systems make way for supportive/educative interventions. However, Susan believes this adaptation to Orem's model will make the most appropriate use of her abilities and is central in helping Victoria to gain more self-care skills.

Expected outcomes

Following many individual sessions in Victoria's home and a visit to the local town, Victoria and Susan agree to try to achieve the following goals:

- identify the likely factors influencing her anxiety;
- identify possible situations which may lead to feelings of unease or anxiety;
- identify thoughts prior to an anxiety attack, and determine whether those thoughts are rational or not, and whether they are useful to problem-solving;
- be aware that anxiety is an important and powerful human emotion, but is temporary and will dissipate;
- identify and utilise appropriate support systems;
- be able to manage interactions with other people without experiencing anxiety;

110

- gain greater confidence to perform activities previously thought impossible.

INTERVENTIONS

A key aspect of Victoria's care is the development of a therapeutic relationship with Susan. Following their initial meeting, Victoria is prepared to meet Susan by herself, and feels more comfortable talking about herself. In fact, she confides to Susan that there have been few instances in her life when anybody has wanted to listen to her, or when she has had something she really wanted to say. Susan is very aware that Victoria can be relaxed when she is in her own home and that anxiety-provoking stimuli can come from a variety of sources quite unexpectedly. Susan is keen to let Victoria know she is aware that anxiety can be a very frightening and disturbing event and that she takes her problems seriously. At all times Susan maintains a quiet and unassuming manner. She is also a careful and respectful listener, and allows Victoria to do much of the talking; this helps develop a working relationship between the two of them.

The role of the physical environment is a key issue for Victoria. When in familiar or controlled settings, anxiety problems are rarely experienced; Victoria claims that it is only when events occur in an unfamiliar environment that there are difficulties. This is important as Orem views the environment as being particularly important to the continued development of an individual. Susan is quick to present the familiar to Victoria at times when she is talking about potentially anxiety-provoking situations. During these times, a soft and lower pitch of voice helps Victoria respond to questions which are potentially stressful to answer.

Susan encourages Victoria to talk about her current situation and her anxieties. In particular a great deal of time is spent in allowing Victoria to identify and explore the threats and anxieties she experiences. Through this approach Victoria may be able to identify events or situations that are likely to be anxiety-provoking and to avoid them if appropriate. Susan helps Victoria to see that in an anxiety state it becomes increasingly difficult to make judgements, take decisions and remember details of conversation and events.

As Victoria starts to feel more comfortable talking about her life and anxieties, Susan instigates a programme of mental exercises (Lewis *et al.* 1989) to help Victoria try to manage her anxiety. These involve Victoria questioning herself about whether a thought is rational or not whenever she is beginning to feel 'uneasy' about a situation. Sometimes Victoria has a warning that she is about to become anxious, at other times she gets none. These exercises may help when there is time to question feelings and experiences.

Coupled with these mental exercises, Susan suggests that Victoria attempt to take on a more positive attitude towards herself; she rarely comments on her own self-image or feelings of worth. Victoria is encouraged to remember that she has experienced difficult situations before and lived through them, and that nothing has occurred as a result of them; she has not fainted, for example, even though she has felt she would. Susan reminds her further that she still has great importance as a mother and grandmother, particularly as her eldest grandson now asks to see and play with her.

Breathing techniques are also taught to Victoria to help keep control of her anxiety. Focusing on breathing rather than on the anxiety may reduce the likelihood of anxiety building up (Knowles 1981). Specifically, it is suggested that she inhale and hold her breath for a couple of seconds before exhaling. Susan tells Victoria she realises that an anxiety state is a particularly uncomfortable experience and that there is a feeling of loss of control. Some of the interventions being developed and adopted by Susan are aimed at giving Victoria more control over her life and aspects of her environment.

The use of imaging has been discussed with Victoria. The aim here is to allow Victoria to suggest to herself that she can be successful in meeting challenging situations. Victoria is asked not to worry about an anxiety-provoking situation or the anxiety she experiences but to look at the situation and 'review' the scenario such that the outcome is more positive and less unpleasant for her (Helmstetter 1987). During these times, Victoria is asked to talk her way through the scenario to clarify problem situations, and plan how she can deal with them.

In addition to these techniques, Susan recommends some behavioural interventions. In particular, Victoria and Susan will go into town together for exposure to situations which Victoria needs to manage if she is to be socially active. A visit to the bank, using a cash dispenser and using a telephone box are some of the activities Susan suggests.

The use of these behavioural interventions is particularly important in managing the self-care requisites of a balance between solitude and social interaction and the promotion of normacy. Victoria lacks self-confidence and is not assertive; she is sensitive to negative comments and criticism in general. In fact, she has feelings of being inferior as well as her practical difficulty in communicating with new people and her poor handwriting ability. The combination of all these problems may have led to Victoria having limited social activity and to her difficulty in making decisions.

EVALUATION

Following six weeks of working with Susan, meeting three or four times a week, Victoria has started to develop insight into her difficulties. She wants to be able to be more self-sufficient and to manage her self-care without the anxiety attacks she has when faced with new and potentially threatening situations. She is also keen to take Susan's advice.

Victoria has been increasingly happy to talk to Susan about issues which up until now she has not discussed with anyone else, particularly in terms of her marriage to Michael. She does become tearful at times when talking about him; she obviously misses him a great deal. Following further discussions, Victoria is becoming a little more insightful and realistic about her feelings for him. She views her married life as relatively happy, although she does consider some years as being 'wasted' when she first moved out of her home town. She also regrets not being at home when her parents and Joe died; all three deaths were sudden and she was totally unprepared.

As for Michael, she talks favourably of him most of the time. She views him as a good husband who provided well for James and herself. Yet she is beginning to become more honest about her marriage to Michael. While not prepared to say critical things about him, she does acknowledge that things could have been different. She would have liked to have been more involved in family finances and the taking of major decisions. Michael also had the annoying habit, she can now admit, of starting many jobs around the house but finishing few of them. Victoria says she feels 'relieved' to talk to Susan about these things.

As part of the evaluation of their care plan, Susan wants to know how Victoria views the relative success of the techniques she has been taught to help manage anxiety. Victoria is keen to try to think through some of the mental exercises suggested by Susan; these however, have been very difficult for her. She is unsure what a rational or non-rational fear is. She realises it can be completely 'normal' to have fear of the unknown, and that fear is sometimes an important physiological response. She feels that she cannot make a clear distinction between what is and what is not rational.

She expresses similar concerns and difficulties managing other mental exercises when she feels anxiety occurring. She confides to Susan, 'I feel so worried about the anxiety and what I might do that I can't think calmly about what's happening.' She has not been able to develop a mental scenario of how her experience could be viewed in an altogether more positive light. She just wants to remove herself from the source of anxiety.

The breathing exercises have helped in some instances of mild anxiety and when Victoria has had some warning of impending concern. She says that it gives her sufficient time to leave a situation and so avoid a 'full-blown' anxiety attack. This has made her feel more in control of her life.

Susan's plan was that Victoria should have learned some of these anxiety-reduction techniques prior to going into town. This, to some extent, has been achieved. Victoria and Susan have therefore gone to the local town on several occasions and have attempted to go together to places which have, in the past, been of concern to Victoria, including the bank, a telephone box, and the town council offices where Victoria needed to talk to someone about her local taxes. Provided someone is with her, Victoria is able to go into these places and deal with her affairs. She functions quite well, in Susan's opinion.

The frequency of Susan's meetings with Victoria, initially three or four times per week, has gradually been tapered off; Susan now sees her only once a week. They agree to have a meeting to discuss how Victoria feels she is managing. At this meeting, Victoria confides that even though she knows much of her fear and anxiety is probably irrational, it is still very real to her. She also says that while the mental techniques sometimes help, her best way of managing her concerns is to avoid the unfamiliar, though she realises this is difficult to achieve.

Victoria does admit, however, to trying new techniques to overcome some of her anxieties. She did, for example, start using direct-debit methods at the bank to avoid having to deal with staff when paying bills in person. While she did need the help of a neighbour to achieve this, she feels quite proud that she has found a solution to one of her difficulties, if not the underlying problem.

Some actions she has not attempted and she says she could not consider doing them by herself, even with the knowledge and insight she has of her condition and the techniques she has learned to use.

These include going anywhere by train, where a spate of minor train accidents and muggings have set real fear in her mind; she uses similar excuses for not travelling by coach. Due to job and other commitments, her son and his family are not able to see her as often as she would like them to visit. Her inability to use public transport has, therefore, caused her some anguish, because without being able to travel she cannot see her son and grandchildren as much as she would like.

Progress

It has now been several months since Victoria first came under community psychiatric care. The initial plans for Victoria's care were aimed at making her more aware of the nature of anxiety, to provide a range of techniques (both mental and physical) to manage anxiety, and to enable her to manage more self-care aspects of her life without the concern for anxiety. Following extensive discussions between Victoria and Susan, they both agree that the improvements, though real, have fallen short of their initial hopes. Victoria has not been able to use the techniques she has practised to manage anxiety when it occurs. Perhaps more importantly, it is the fear of anxiety which has been particularly problematic. Victoria has an overpowering need to avoid the *risk* of anxiety even though she realises that most of it could be irrational and that no physical harm comes to her. This situation has continued to cause her distress. She wants to be able to travel by herself, to see her friends and family, but the risks for her are too great. As she says, 'Whatever I try I can't win. I feel bad that I can't travel to see my son and I feel bad when I think about travelling'.

Victoria's response over the past months has been to be very receptive to Susan's suggestions and ideas and to develop a greater knowledge about the nature of her difficulties and possible ways to manage them. But this knowledge by itself has not been enough. She has retained many of the behaviours she was using to avoid anxiety before she met Susan. The same dilemmas are present. Victoria can manage to perform most self-care activities which involve her with the familiar, provided it is within her home town. Once she steps outside these boundaries, difficulties occur.

Susan realises that the aims agreed between the two some months earlier were probably too ambitious, yet the time spent together has certainly not been a complete waste. She continues to believe that a supportive/educative nursing system is the appropriate starting point and that further work should follow this approach. Victoria believes that even though she cannot do many of the things she wants to, working with Susan has helped her view her life in a different way, and she has been able to express views and opinions she previously had not been able to. It is time for Victoria and Susan to rethink their strategies.

Following renewed discussions between them, new areas of exploration have been identified. Most important are Victoria's feelings and attitudes towards her husband and his death. Grief for the loss of a loved one can take many forms and can be an extremely traumatic experience (Barry 1984; Bowlby 1961; Kubler-Ross 1975). This aspect of Victoria's life must become the focus of Susan's attention.

Currently they are exploring issues surrounding Michael, their marriage, and his death. Victoria wants to become more involved in living, yet her anxieties are still preventing her from managing key universal and developmental self-care requisites.

FOLLOW-UP WORK

Questions

1 Using Orem's model in the way suggested in this care study requires the nurse to move away from the physical aspects of care, towards more psychosocial and developmental concerns. Consider the following aspects of Orem's work.

   (a) Developmental self-care requisites are sometimes difficult to identify and to incorporate into a care plan. If, following an assessment, you identified a possible developmental self-care problem, such as educational or social deprivation, how would you use that information in your care plan? How could you validate your findings or suspicions?

   (b) This care study illustrated the importance of considering family events and the notion of 'normal' behaviours and reactions to occurrences. How would you as a nurse determine whether a response or behaviour could be considered, in the widest possible sense, 'normal'? How might culture influence your decisions? What role does the client have in your assessment?

116

2 Victoria has been exhibiting many instances of avoiding situations which she believes to be threatening or anxiety-provoking. This is particularly important considering her self-care limitation of difficulty with social interaction. Consider the following:

(a) Is avoidance behaviour always to be refrained from?
(b) In what instances might avoidance be a 'healthy' response to a situation?
(c) What role do you think avoidance may have in an individual's decision to seek or not to seek assistance from suitably qualified individuals in meeting self-care demands?

Activities

Orem considers that observational skills are an essential component of a nurse's skill repertoire. Anxiety can be brought about by any number of things. Consider your experiences both as a nurse and within the community when addressing the following:

- What range of responses can an individual elicit during times of anxiety?
- What problems are there in measuring, quantifying or assessing anxiety?
- What role can cultural difference play in your determinations?
- How could you validate your findings?

PART III

Critique of the model

CHAPTER EIGHT

Evaluation

INTRODUCTION

In Part II, Orem's model of nursing was used in a variety of settings to assess, plan, implement and evaluate patient care. It is hoped that these readings and exercises, coupled with your own nursing experiences, have given you some familiarity with the model. Perhaps you have even started to use it in planning the care of patients. Whatever your level of exposure, you are no doubt starting to formulate your own views. Does Orem actually help in planning care? What are the strengths and weaknesses of her model? How can the model work in specific areas of practice?

This section will put Dorothea Orem's views of nursing, as exemplified in her model, into a wider perspective, and provide a framework for a critical examination of the model. (Incidentally, the approach suggested here to analyse Orem can readily be adapted to other models.) There is no simple answer to whether Orem's model is inherently 'good' or 'bad', but this framework may help you to make your own decision.

AN OVERVIEW OF OREM'S MODEL

There can be little doubt that Dorothea Orem's model of nursing has made a great impact on the nursing profession. The model is used by many American universities and colleges as the conceptual framework underpinning undergraduate nurse education, and it is also studied in the UK and Holland, as well as other European countries. But as well as influencing academic thinking about nursing, the model has also made a significant impact upon nursing practice. Nurses are using Orem's model as a foundation for the planning and delivery of patient care.

It is important, however, to look critically at some of the reasons for this implementation. Certainly the model offers an immediate utility for nurses and patient care. While there may be some difficulties with the language of the model (more will be said on this later), the notion of nursing practice being a substitute for or supplement to an individual's self-care abilities is immediately understood. Additionally, it can be argued that Orem's ideas are a logical extension of some of the ideas espoused by Florence Nightingale and Virginia Henderson, and are thus central to nursing's primary concern for patient care.

Despite the similarities with other great nursing thinkers, there are other reasons why Orem has become both known and popular in this country. One of the many changes in nurse education has been a move away from the medical-model approach to patient care. Increasingly, nursing is focusing its attentions on issues of promoting health. Meleis (1985) has suggested that in moving from a medically-orientated to a health-orientated perspective of care, nurses have required and utilised both a 'needs' and a 'functional' approach to their practice: Orem's model offers both, and therefore eases the transition process.

At the same time, however, the model does not attempt to break all links with nursing's deep-seated history of having its education rooted within a medical orientation. As Johnson (1983) observes, Orem makes no attempt to reject the medical perspective but chooses to integrate it into the model. In fact there are many instances where the model adopts medical language to describe key aspects of Orem's ideas, notably in the use of the terms 'patient' and 'diagnosis'. This foundation within a familiar educational tradition has undoubtedly contributed to the model's popularity. Orem is not alone here; it can be argued, for instance, that the Roper–Logan–Tierney model (1986) has gained popularity for similar reasons.

Nursing models must, however, be viewed outside the realm of an academic setting: how can they be examined and utilised in the real world of nursing practice? In the case of Orem's model by far the greatest area of implementation has been within hospitals, with clients who are obviously experiencing health problems: in view of the model's 'medical' tendencies, this is hardly surprising. In addition the model as a whole has its foundation rooted in institutional care and the individual. This in itself may be an important feature to consider when deciding which model to examine and to utilise in practice, particularly for those nurses who see their primary role as 'caring for the sick'. Orem's model will, by its very nature, appeal to some nurses because of its medically-orientated language and its immediate relevance to hospital-based nursing care, which still forms an essential part of a nurse's training.

AN EVALUATION FRAMEWORK

As well as examining the background to the popularity of the model, consideration must be given to a more critical examination, and to 'reading between the lines' of the model. Given the proliferation of nursing models within the past twenty years, nurses need a frame of reference in which to assess the relative contributions of the differing models to nursing practice, research and knowledge.

Several authors have presented schemes for evaluating nursing models (Walker and Avant 1983; Fawcett 1984; Stevens 1984). Each provides a well-argued approach to discussing theories and models to permit practising nurses to make a more informed choice about the use of models and to help identify relative strengths and weaknesses. Such evaluations can also form the basis of a much more academic study of nursing and knowledge-building.

The purpose of this section is to concentrate on evaluating Orem's model from the perspective of action – does it facilitate the process of nursing? The following headings, which serve as a guide to model evaluation, are taken primarily from the works of Walker and Avant (1983) and Stevens (1984). These authors have been chosen because of their systematic and logical approach to examining models; this section draws particularly on Stevens's work, which begins by establishing that there can be both external and internal criticism of a model.

External criticism

External criticism, as applied in the following sub-sections, refers to the examination of Orem's work as it relates to the real world of nursing. Essentially, it addresses the question of whether the model works when put into practice. But how is effectiveness defined? The following are some criteria which can be applied to address this question.

Underlying principles

At the heart of any nursing model is the expression of what the theorist perceives to be the nature of nursing, health, a person, and

123

society. One of the key questions to be considered before you can work with a model is the extent to which the theorist's perceptions are congruent with your own: if you cannot abide by the underlying philosophy of the model, it will be difficult to make it the basis for practice.

Put simply, the model itself is constructed around a series of assumptions or premises which are linked together in a logical way to form the model. An essential component of model evaluation is consideration of these assumptions.

The nature of man   Orem makes some major assumptions about the nature of man. She proposes that a healthy individual is self-caring, knows when he is in need of assistance, can actually seek information and understand it when given, and is then willing to act upon it. Thus, the emphasis is on individual self-care deficits rather than on the biopsychosocial being. In fact, there are many people within our society who cannot fulfil Orem's requirements, not because of religious or cultural differences, but because of their individual differences. For example, they may not have the language skills that would enable them to seek help. Yet Orem also recognises that the methods an individual uses to manage self-care needs are culturally based, and that there is no single way to meet self-care demands.

One of the key steps in entering any health-care system is that the individual (unless unconscious) must perceive that he has a need for assistance. In this view, it is up to individuals to know about themselves and to recognise when help is needed. Again this is a rational stance. There are many instances when people are experiencing changes in their health yet for a variety of reasons choose not to seek help. Some conditions may be expected to resolve themselves without nursing intervention; while fear, peer pressure, and practicalities such as transportation and cost may all interfere with an individual's decision to seek advice.

Orem also places the responsibility on the individual to acquire the necessary information and skills to manage his own health needs or to seek assistance and advice from others. This in itself is a complicated set of behaviours; learning how to find information can itself be difficult and off-putting. In most areas of education and nurse training, one of the first skills to be taught is that of information retrieval! To find information or to seek advice requires many skills; language, social skills and intellectual abilities feature prominently in this process. Again, not all members of society will have these abilities sufficiently developed to manage this process effectively.

A further assumption made by Orem about man is that the performance of self-care behaviours is a deliberate and calculated action based upon an individual's knowledge and skills repertoire. The essential point here is that of an individual's free will. Orem assumes that an individual has the ability to make choices. There will, however, be instances when one is temporarily unable to make decisions or choices, or when the decision taken is not appropriate. Anxiety, fear or other concerns might take a higher priority than individual needs.

Finally, Orem suggests that individuals will investigate and develop ways to meet known self-care demands. This may require highly developed physical or intellectual skills, which not everyone will possess at all times.

What emerges from this is a series of responsibilities placed upon us to manage our own self-care needs. Orem takes as her starting point an individual who has highly developed language, social and information retrieval skills, as well as the ability to make informed decisions. It follows that a large number of people within our society may not have all the requisite skills to manage their own self-care needs. They will require assistance to enter into a health-care system.

The nature of nursing Orem's model has a special place in the nursing literature because of its attempts to define the boundaries of nursing: when it is appropriate for nursing care to be initiated and when nursing care ends. While this is important, it does give rise to some anomalies: if the model were adopted *de facto* and individuals had no self-care deficits, would nursing have any purpose? This may at first glance preclude any health-promotion role for nursing, but Orem does in fact advocate that health promotion is an important role for nursing.

Orem also raises vital issues about the nature of nursing which challenge the profession today. She makes a clear distinction between 'professional' and 'technical' acts of nursing, which implies a distinction also between the roles and responsibilities of qualified nursing staff and their aides, the assistants or technicians who 'supply nursing'. This distinction rests on education and the moral nature of nursing: nurses must be able to ask and to answer the question, is this act right for the patient? Orem suggests that if assistants are employed to supply nursing services, they should have a dependent-care type of relationship with a professional nurse.

Orem also raises the issues of professional nurse education. She is concerned that there are many qualified nurses who are 'intellectually impoverished' in their professional endeavours at a time when there is an enormous growth in knowledge about health and health-related issues. Individuals entering nursing must learn to combine the roles of being both a student of nursing practice and a nursing scholar. Such concerns have influenced the development of Project 2000 courses in this country.

The nature of health   In keeping with many other aspects of her model, Orem, by defining health in terms of structural and functional soundness and wholeness, relies heavily on a medical model which is based on the absence of signs and symptoms. Health is conceptualised in relation to self-care deficits. Within the nursing process, this forms the primary focus of the nursing function of assessment using self-care requisites.

While this may seem narrow in focus, Orem has attempted in the 1991 edition of her model to extend the boundaries of health to include primary, secondary and tertiary levels of prevention. These notions of prevention can work well provided that the individual is under legitimate nursing care. Orem, in fact, directs nurses to use the universal self-care requisite of the prevention of hazards to life, human functioning and well-being to detail preventive aspects of nursing care. Problems may arise when an individual chooses not to enter into a therapeutic relationship with nursing staff.

The nature of the environment   The least well articulated components of Orem's model are those of the nature of the environment and of the interactions between individuals and the environment. What does emerge is that Orem considers that the environment, both in a physical form and in a psychosocial form, can influence an individual's development. From these general relationships it is possible to hypothesise that poor housing or perhaps the death of a family member can influence human development. This may in turn lead to difficulties in meeting self-care requirements. A word of caution here, however: to develop Orem's model to this level of sophistication requires considerable conceptual clarification and research. Much more attention needs to be focused on this neglected area of the model.

Utility

Having considered the fundamental assumptions of the model, the utilisation of the model must be examined: does the model facilitate nursing practice?

Orem, in keeping with most other nursing theorists, poses problems for the reader by her use of language. (Overcoming this problem has been a key reason for the Nursing Models in Action series of books.) Nurses are obliged to grapple with a new and often bewildering vocabulary before they can examine the model's utility in practice. Also, some models may be accused of being too esoteric for nursing practice of today.

General care issues   The following are some general observations about aspects of the model, beginning with the process of assessment. The issues to be raised here are particularly relevant to some of the care plans presented in Part II of this book. Throughout this section you are encouraged to draw upon your reading of those care plans and on your own discussions or experiences with Orem's model to supplement the text.

Orem requires the nurse undertaking the assessment of a patient to consider three categories of self-care requisites: universal, developmental and health-deviation. One of the initial concerns with almost all nursing models is that of being comprehensive – given a framework for assessment, are there 'categories' or 'compartments' in keeping with the structure of the model in which to enter all the data collected? Once you have become familiar with the model's language, it must be clear how assessment data should be recorded and organised.

In Orem's model, the universal self-care requisites offer eight broad categories for entering primarily 'physical' data. While there is an opportunity for psychosocial material to be considered, the emphasis is clearly on the behaviours necessary to maintain life. Orem does not specifically indicate how particular data should be associated with particular universal self-care requisites; this can be problematic. Where, for example, should pain and pain relief be documented? Likewise, anxiety and fear, essential considerations in any nursing assessment, are not obviously linked to one specific requisite. Only with experience, discussion and confidence in the model will nurses overcome these potential difficulties. However, while acknowledging these possible shortcomings, it is important to stress that a vital component of any nursing model is its ability to assist thinking and the exploration of patient care issues.

This illustrates an important issue which faces most nursing models, namely that few are developed sufficiently to meet all nursing care circumstances. In fact, Orem admits that it is up to the nurse to 'use' the model in any way which facilitates nursing practice. While this is an important recognition by Orem, it does pose problems. Without specific guidelines it is easy to imagine that staff will hold a multitude of different 'perceptions' of the model, which may hamper continuity of care. While the model can stimulate new thinking and ideas about care, and thus about the variety of situations in which the model can be applied, key concepts must be understood in the same way by all those using, reviewing, or researching Orem-based care.

The other risk in allowing the proliferation of potentially different approaches to Orem – or to any other model for that matter – is that the essential structure and philosophy of the model may be lost to utilitarianism. That is, Orem's model may become simply a mechanism for charting, rather than a unique way of viewing the needs of patients and the special nurse–patient relationship.

Similar concerns can be voiced about developmental and health-deviation self-care requisites. A common observation about these requisites is that frequently they are either overlooked or incompletely assessed. With the concentration on universal requisites, aspects of special needs associated with a developmental stage, such as pregnancy or infancy, can be forgotten. It is important to remember that the process of learning self-care is itself developmental, and can therefore be influenced by a wide range of factors. The impact of educational deprivation, economic status and living conditions on self-care abilities is rarely considered. Frequently this is simply because there are few known facts or observable data to record. How does a nurse attempt to determine the impact of poor housing on an individual's ability to be self-caring?

Health-deviation self-care requisites pose similar concerns in that they require longitudinal assessment. To verify a piece of assessment data or to determine whether an intervention has been 'successful' can take a considerable period of time, longer than the client's likely contact with nursing care. For example, following an amputation or a burn, how long will it take to determine whether the individual can adapt, or has adapted, to his situation and confirm that he is continuing his personal development? It seems unlikely in the acute-care sector that every patient will be followed closely enough to answer these types of questions.

Psychiatry Nursing models have been developed primarily in the medical/surgical sector of health care: they have seldom been applied in the psychiatric setting. Dashiff (1988) suggests this is due to four factors: unfamiliarity of language and cumbersome terminology; relatively few courses in psychiatric nursing dealing with nursing models; psychiatric nurses preferring to use the ideas and theories from other mental-health disciplines rather than nursing; and few mental-health settings working from a nursing conceptual framework or having leaders who would act as nursing theory role-models.

Dashiff's ideas probably contain truth, and there are some genuine concerns about Orem's perceptions of man in relation to the mental-health setting. Orem's work centres on the contractual relationship between patient and nurse, essentially a contract between a nurse and a client who can put a rational value on their own health. The general objection to using models like Orem's in the mental-health setting is summarised by Moscovitz (1984): arguing from a psychoanalytical perspective, she suggests that Orem's model, because it focuses on value judgements and rational decision-making, neglects the role of unconscious and irrational aspects of an individual's behaviour. The case is cited of the client who, rather than wishing to be independent, needs to be nurtured: Orem's model has conceptual difficulty in dealing with this situation. Moscovitz goes on to suggest that there is always the likelihood of internal resistance to accepting nursing help because of a client's need to defend himself against anxiety and fear. In these situations, the client may have 'inner' conflict to which the nurse under Orem's model can respond only with 'external' modalities of care, such as doing for and assisting. Similar difficulties could occur when working with clients who have severe learning disabilities: Orem fails to clarify the care that can be offered to these groups of clients, generally relegating their care to the wholly compensatory system of care without exploring alternative strategies.

Despite these arguments, however, Orem does recognise both the importance of internal and unconscious behaviours and that a client's ability to take deliberate self-care action could be interfered with by the psychological disturbances which can result in emotional reactions. Managing some internal behaviours permits self-care to take place and is an important aspect of nursing care. From a conceptual perspective, Orem's model *can* therefore have a place in the psychiatric setting; however, few have attempted to explore the possibilities of adopting this model in this context.

Children and others in dependent-care relationships A commonly encountered criticism of Orem's model is that it fails to take account directly of the wishes and needs of those individuals who may not be developmentally able to express themselves, or who are unable to make independent decisions. The nursing care of young children is an example of this. There is in general little discussion of the nurse–patient relationship when the patient is a child. The nursing care of children is generally considered to be a dependent-care relationship, usually one in which the care of the family is central. It is possible that a child's unique needs could go unmet when dealing with complex family relationships. Further, as Melnyk (1983) observes, there is an ambiguity in this situation as the child is not yet his own self-care agent and the healthy parent has no self-care deficits.

Despite these conceptual anomalies, there are many strengths in considering the entire family when a child is in need of health-care assistance. Tadych (1985) proposes that Orem's model can assist in three ways: it can help the family to develop the capacity to view itself as the unit of structure and function; it can foster the development of self-care or dependent-care capabilities; and it can foster the capability to observe and analyse the interrelatedness of therapeutic self-care demands among members of the family and to plan to meet these demands and secure the necessary resources to do so. Essentially, this approach may help the family look more closely at its own dynamics, and can actually help families begin to solve their own problems and difficulties. This occurs when the child is being considered as part of the family, not as a separate individual.

Health promotion Well individuals are becoming an increasingly important aspect of organised health care. Well-women and child clinics are becoming more common in the UK. There is also the important question of the school nurse: Orem fails to deal adequately with this group of nurses. One reason for this is that she is hindered by her definition of nursing care, which focuses on being unable to meet, at the present time, some self-care need. But what is the nurse's role when an individual is healthy and has no self-care deficits? This leaves the issue of health promotion and preventive health care largely unexplored. Yet an essential aspect of nursing care and client education is the development of good health practices for life. The nursing community has realised this ambiguity and is looking at ways of applying Orem's work to the health-promotion aspect of nursing practice (Hill and Smith 1985).

Orem (1991, p.195) does recognise the importance of primary, secondary and tertiary levels of prevention, and that these have implications for the life, health and effective living of the patient; but for a nurse to assist there must already be a nurse–patient interaction, or a nursing situation. Orem begins to address this difficulty in saying that if a person is unknowing about issues in health care then nursing has a role in helping that individual to become aware of them. This may, conceptually at least, expand the potential sphere of nursing influence.

Orem and the nursing process   Orem utilises the familiar framework of the nursing process to organise the activities of nursing. Although she actually states that the technologic-professional aspects of the nursing process consists of four operations designated 'diagnostic', 'prescriptive', 'regulation or treatment' and 'control', these four are similar to the 'traditional' approach of assessing, planning, intervening and evaluating care commonly seen in the UK.

The use of the nursing system – that is, deciding whether care should be wholly compensatory, partly compensatory or supportive/ educative – can cause some practical and philosophical difficulties. The reality is that it can be extremely difficult to decide upon a system of care for a patient. It has already been noted that to place an individual in a wholly compensatory nursing system because of physical needs alone, when that person still has some decision-making ability, seems problematic. As a patient's condition improves, the move from wholly to partly compensatory becomes a matter of judgement: the nurse, as Orem intends, must make a decision based upon education and experience.

Conclusion   Orem's model is indeed useful to many aspects of nursing practice but does have some limitations. Nevertheless it is a workable and practice-orientated model. From the increasing volume of literature about the application of Orem's model to care settings in the UK and the care studies in this book, it is clear that the model can be used without major modifications, despite its having been developed in the USA. Irrespective of geographical and cultural issues, Orem remains unique in her attempt to define the boundaries of nursing and nursing practice.

Discrimination

'Discrimination' refers to the ability of a model to differentiate nurses from other health professionals and nursing from other caring or tending acts. When Orem began to develop her model of nursing in the USA, most educational programmes were based upon models more representative of other disciplines such as medicine, psychology and sociology. With Orem's emphasis on moving towards a nursing focus (although it still does have many similarities to a medical-model approach), she has contributed significantly to nursing knowledge by providing an explicit and specific focus for nursing assessment, planning, implementation and evaluation of care. This approach is different from those adopted by other professionals. The greatest strengths of her model can be considered to be the incorporation of the major ideas of self-care for individuals at various levels of health, and a supportive/educative nursing system.

However, the nursing role can still be confused within the Orem model, because of the role of the doctor in the nurse–patient relationship. Orem's basic view of nursing is of the rational adult patient who is able to acknowledge a self-care deficit and who allows the nurse, upon the recommendation of the doctor, to provide nursing care. Taken to its extreme, Orem's model suggests that nursing and the nurse–patient relationship require an external authority to define, initiate and make legitimate nursing practice (Melnyk 1983). There are many aspects of modern nursing practice which permit nursing intervention without the direct authorisation or ultimate supervision of nursing care.

Generalisability

Generalisability is considered to be the range of patients and patient-care situations that can be addressed by the model. The central recipient of Orem's attention is the competent individual able to seek and follow advice from another. This perspective may be appropriate at times, but generally the model does not place sufficient emphasis on the fact that an individual interacts with family and friends as well as with the environment. The nature of these interactions for the adult is not well described. The role of significant others in the organisation of care seems not to have a high priority in care planning. This is in contrast to one dependent-care relationship that is discussed in detail, the one in which the complex role of the child within a family is at the centre of the nursing focus.

The definitions of the three nursing systems – wholly compensatory, partly compensatory and supportive-educative – should provide an approach to care which encompasses all nursing situations. There are, however, some anomalies to consider. What of the individual who has severe physical difficulties yet possesses all his mental faculties? To place this individual in a wholly compensatory nursing system because of his need to have a large number of physical needs met fails to acknowledge his continuing ability to make informed decisions about his own care.

Concerns have also been voiced about the cultural and socio-economic aspects of the model. Fawcett (1984) claims that these issues are largely ignored by Orem. The primary difficulty is that Orem requires the goal of self-care to be met mutually by the patient and the nurse. There are, however, many different cultural perspectives of the sick role which are not compatible with this view.

Research The relationship between a nursing model and nursing research can be a complicated one. (For a more comprehensive review of this subject, see Walker and Avant 1983 and Stevens 1984.) One of the ways in which the nursing community, and indeed the scientific community in general, develops confidence in a model is by conducting research to examine its basic assumptions and claims. There has been some research into Orem's model and the general principles of self-care. The initial work has been to develop instruments to measure a client's involvement with self-care; in particular, Kearney and Fleisher (1979) have described a reliable and valid instrument which assesses an individual's self-care agency. Additionally Kuriansky *et al.* (1976) have developed the Performance Test of Activities of Daily Living (PADL) to measure self-care agency.

It has taken considerable time to develop these tools because of the inherent difficulties of attempting to operationalise, or quantify, complex terms emerging from the model. How do you measure self-care agency? This has not been helped by the internal difficulties of the model (described below). Nevertheless, research into self-care is continuing despite these difficulties, and a selection of reports is indicated in the bibliography of this book. Research is continuing to test the propositions, such as self-care, underlying Orem's model.

Internal criticism

The internal consistency of a model deals with how well its assumptions, concepts and theoretical statements fit together (Stevens 1984). One of the difficulties faced by the reader of Orem is that of being completely clear about the definitions of terms used throughout the model. As well as being problematic from an educational and practice perspective – a great deal of time has to be spent learning and agreeing what each of the components actually means – this also poses difficulty for the researcher. Without agreement on how to use components of the model, inconsistencies in application and investigation are inevitable. This is one of the major internal criticisms of Orem; there is a lack of clarity of concepts. Further, Orem has made little attempt to define her terms in a way that is immediately quantifiable: from a positivistic viewpoint, this gives rise to some very practical concerns. If nurses are not completely clear about the meaning, application and recording of the model's tenets, how is consistency in practice to develop? Despite this criticism, Orem does seem to use terms consistently throughout the model, which is important for the practitioner, the educator and the researcher.

There are many other technical and esoteric aspects of the internal criticism of Orem's model which will not be considered here. For an authoritative in-depth discussion of the internal and external criticism of Orem's model, see Fitzpatrick and Whall (1983) and Feathers (1989).

CONCLUSION

Dorothea Orem's model has made a profound impact on nursing practice, education and administration. Her ideas have made an important contribution in seeking to define the nature and bounds of nursing. While providing a framework to guide and facilitate nursing practice, Orem has devised a workable model for planning care for all those in need of health-care assistance.

In attempting to develop a highly complex structure of inter-related concepts and ideas, there are bound to be inconsistencies and areas of ambiguity. It has been noted that Orem is not alone in failing to adequately define or quantify some of her ideas. What is important is that a framework for practice has been put into nursing's domain to use as nurses see fit. As Melnyk (1983) believes, to implement Orem's (or any other) model scrupulously and without question would limit nursing practice to protocol, regulations and procedures all specified by the doctor. This is far removed from Orem's vision. Nursing and nurses must use this model in whatever way they see fit, to facilitate practice, research and the development of new knowledge.

When considering the internal consistency of a model there is often a broad consensus of agreement; it is not too difficult to agree if a definition is unworkable or if there is a logical fallacy in the way concepts are used. The same cannot be said for the external criticism of a model, as this touches upon much wider issues of professional practice and a variety of settings. As a result, you may not agree with all the issues raised in this evaluation, but you may find them useful when discussing or using this, or any other, model. Orem's model can, when understood, be sensibly applied to a wide range of practices, but it will take imagination and a commitment in its use to strive for the highest standards of nursing care.

GLOSSARY

This glossary comprises extracts from the 4th edition (1991) of Dorothea Orem's *Nursing: Concepts and Practice* (pp. 361–6), reprinted with the permission of Mosby Year Book Inc., Missouri.

agency   The power to engage in action to achieve specific goals.

dependent care   The practice of activities that responsible maturing and mature persons initiate and perform on behalf of socially dependent persons for some time on a continuing basis in order to maintain their lives and contribute to their health and well-being.

dependent-care agency   The developed and developing capabilities of persons to know and meet the therapeutic self-care demands of persons socially dependent on them or to regulate the development or exercise of these persons' self-care agency.

dependent-care agent   A maturing adolescent or adult who accepts and fulfills the responsibility to know and meet the therapeutic self-care demand of relevant others who are socially dependent on them or to regulate the development or exercise of these persons' self-care agency.

health   A descriptor of living things with respect to their structural and functional wholeness and soundness.

nursing agency   The developed capabilities of persons educated as nurses that empower them to represent themselves as nurses and within the frame of a legitimate interpersonal relationship to act, to know, and to help persons in such relationships to meet their therapeutic self-care demands and to regulate the development or exercise of their self-care agency.

nursing diagnosis   A deliberate process through which nurses in nursing practice situations carefully examine and analyze facts and judgments about persons who are their patients, and about properties and activities of these persons, to explain and state the nature and causes of their therapeutic self-care demands; the state of development, the operability and adequacy of their self-care agency; and the presence and extent of self-care deficits existent or projected.

nursing design   A professional function performed both before and after nursing diagnosis and prescription through which nurses, on the basis of reflective practical judgments about existent conditions, synthesize concrete situational elements into orderly relations to structure operational units. The purpose of nursing design is to provide guides for achieving needed and foreseen results in the production of nursing toward the achievement of nursing goals; the units taken together constitute the pattern to guide the production of nursing.

nursing prescription   A deliberate action process through which nurses make practical judgments about what can and should be done to meet their patients' particularized self-care requisites and to regulate the exercise or development of their self-care agency under existent or projected changed conditions and circumstances.

nursing regulation or treatment   Nurses' use of valid and reliable measures to continuously meet their patients' particularized self-care requisites in order to keep their functioning and development within ranges compatible with life and with normal functioning and development; it also includes use of measures to ensure that patients' developed or potential powers of self-care agency are protected and the exercise or development of self-care agency regulated.

nursing systems   Series and sequences of deliberate practical actions of nurses performed at times in coordination with actions of their patients to know and meet components of their patients' therapeutic self-care demands to protect and regulate the exercise or development of patients' self-care agency.

self-care   The practice of activities that maturing and mature persons initiate and perform, within time frames, on their own behalf in the interests of maintaining life, healthful functioning, continuing personal development, and well-being.

self-care agency   The complex acquired ability of mature and maturing persons to know and meet their continuing requirements for deliberate, purposive action to regulate their own human functioning and development.

self-care deficit   A relation between the human properties therapeutic self-care demand and self-care agency in which constituent developed self-care capabilities within self-care agency are not operable or not adequate for knowing and meeting some or all components of the existent or projected therapeutic self-care demand.

self-care requisite   A formulated and expressed insight about actions to be performed that are known or hypothesized to be necessary in the regulation of an aspect(s) of human functioning and development continuously or under specified conditions and circumstances. A formulated self-care requisite names (1) the factor to be controlled or managed to keep an aspect(s) of human functioning and development within norms compatible with life and health and personal well-being and (2) the nature of the required action. Formulated and expressed self-care requisite

137

constitutes the formalized purposes of self-care. They are the reasons for which self-care is undertaken; they express the intended or desired results – the goals of self-care.

therapeutic self-care demand The summation of care measures necessary at specific times or over a duration of time for meeting all of an individual's known self-care requisites particularized for existent conditions and circumstances using methods appropriate for (1) controlling or managing factors identified in the requisites the values of which are regulatory of human functioning, for example, sufficiency of air, water, food; and (2) fulfilling the activity element of the requisite, for example, maintenance, promotion, prevention, and provision.

Chapter 1

Aggleton, P. and Chalmers, H. 1986. *Nursing Models and the Nursing Process*. Basingstoke: Macmillan.

Orem, D. E. 1991. *Nursing: Concepts of Practice*, 4th edn. New York: McGraw-Hill.

Orem, D. E. and Taylor, S. G. 1986. Orem's general theory of nursing. In Winstead-Fry, (ed.), *Case Studies in Nursing Theory*. New York: National League of Nursing.

Chapter 2

Reilly, D. E. and Oermann, M. 1985. *The Clinical Field: its use in nursing education*. Norwalk, Connecticut: Appleton-Century-Crofts.

Chapter 4

Backscheider, J. E. 1974. Self-care requirements, self-care capabilities and nursing systems in the diabetic nurse management clinic. *American Journal of Public Health* **64**(12), 1138–1146.

Fitzgerald, S. 1980. Utilizing Orem's self-care nursing model in designing an educational program for the diabetic. *Topics in Clinical Nursing: education for self-care* **2**(2), 57–65.

Porth, C. M. 1986. *Pathophysiology: concepts of altered health states*. New York: Lippincott.

Chapter 5

Billings, D. M. and Stokes, L. S. 1987. *Medical-Surgical Nursing*. St. Louis: Mosby.

Porth, C. M. 1986. *Pathophysiology: concepts of altered health states*. New York: Lippincott.

Chapter 6

Erikson, E. H. 1963. *Childhood and Society*. New York: Norton.
Olds, S. W. and Papalia, D. E. 1986. *Human Development*. New York: McGraw-Hill.
Orem, D. E. 1991. *Nursing: Concepts of Practice*. 4th edn. New York: McGraw-Hill.
Piaget, J. 1952. *The Origins of Intelligence in Children*. New York: International Universities Press.

Chapter 7

Barry, P. D. 1984. *Psychosocial Nursing Assessment and Intervention*. New York: Lippincott.
Bowlby, J. 1961. Processes of mourning. *International Journal of Psychoanalysis* **42**, 317.
Helmstetter, S. 1987. *The Self-Talk Solution*. New York: William Morrow.
Knowles, R. D. 1981. Managing anxiety. *American Journal of Nursing* **81**, 110–11.
Kubler-Ross, E. 1975. *Death: the final stage of growth*. New Jersey: Prentice-Hall.
Lewis, S., Grainger, R. D. K., McDowell, W. A., Gregory, R. J., and Messner, R. L. 1989. *Manual of Psychosocial Nursing Interventions*. **Location:** Saunders.

Chapter 8

Dashiff, C. J. 1988. Theory development in psychiatric-mental health nursing: an analysis of Orem's Theory. *Archives of Psychiatric Nursing* **2**(6), 366–72.
Fawcett, J. 1984. *Analysis and Evaluation of Conceptual Models of Nursing*. Philadephia: Davis.
Feathers, R. L. 1989. Orem's self-care nursing theory. In Riehl-Sisca, J. (ed.), *Conceptual Models for Nursing Practice*, 3rd edn. (pp. 359–68). Norwalk, Connecticut: Appleton & Lange.
Fitzpatrick, J. and Whall, A. L. 1983. *Conceptual Models of Nursing: analysis and application*. Bowie, Maryland: Robert J. Brady.
Hill, L. and Smith, N. 1985. *Self-Care Nursing*. New Jersey: Prentice-Hall.
Johnston, R. L. 1983. Orem self-care model of nursing. In Fitzpatrick and Whall 1983 op. cit.

Kearney, B. Y. and Fleischer, B. J. 1979. Development of an instrument to measure exercise of self-care agency. *Research in Nursing and Health* **2**(1), 25–34.

Kuriansky, J., Gurland, B., Fleiss, J., and Cowan, D. 1976. The assessment of self-care capacity in geriatric psychiatric patients by objective and subjective methods. *Journal of Clinical Psychology* **32**, 95–102.

Meleis, A. I. 1985. *Theoretical Nursing: development and progress*. New York: Lippincott.

Melnyk, K. A. M. 1983. The process of theory analysis: an examination of the nursing theory of Dorothea E. Orem. *Nursing Research* **32**(3), 170–4.

Moscovitz, A. O. 1984. Orem's theory as applied to psychiatric nursing. *Perspectives in Psychiatric Care* **22**, 36–8.

Orem, D. E. 1985. *Nursing: Concepts of Practice*, 3rd edn. New York: McGraw-Hill.

Orem, D. E. 1991. *Nursing: Concepts of Practice*, 4th edn. New York: McGraw-Hill.

Roper, N., Logan, W. and Tierney, A. 1986. *The Elements of Nursing*. Edinburgh: Churchill Livingstone.

Stevens, B. 1984. *Nursing Theory: analysis, application and evaluation*, 2nd edn. Boston: Little, Brown.

Tadych, R. 1985. Nursing in multiperson units: the family. In Sisca, J. R. (ed.), *The science and art of self-care* (pp. 54–8). Norwalk, Connecticut: Appleton-Century-Crofts.

Walker, L. and Avant, K. 1983. *Strategies for Theory Construction in Nursing*. Norwalk, Connecticut: Appleton-Century-Crofts.

The following works can be used to supplement this text, and to give other examples of how Orem's model can be applied in a variety of clinical, managerial and educational settings. Those titles marked with an asterisk (*) are particularly important and useful works.

Theory and nursing models

Aggleton, P. and Chalmers, H. 1985. Models and theories: Orem's self-care model (Part 5). *Nursing Times* **81**(1), 36–9.

*Aggleton, P. and Chalmers, H. 1986. *Nursing Models and the Nursing Process*. London: Macmillan.

Chapman, P. 1984. Specifics and generalities: a critical examination of two nursing models ... Orem's and Preisner's. *Nurse Education Today* **4**(6), 141–4.

Chavasse, J. M. 1987. A comparison of three models of nursing. *Nurse Education Today* **7**(4), 177–86.

Coleman, L. J. 1980. Orem's self-care concept of nursing. In Riehl, J. P. and Roy, C., (eds), *Conceptual Models for Nursing Practice*, 2nd edn (pp. 314–28). New York: Appleton-Century-Crofts.

Dickson, G. L. and Lee-Villasenor, H. 1982. Nursing theory and practice: a self-care approach. *Advances in Nursing Science* **5**, 29–40.

Duffey, M. and Muhlenkamp, A. 1974. A framework for theory analysis. *Nursing Outlook* **22**, 570–4.

*Fawcett, J. 1984. *Analysis and Evaluation of Conceptual Models of Nursing*. Philadephia: Davis.

*Feathers, R. L. 1989. Orem's self-care nursing theory. In Riehl-Sisca, J. (ed.), *Conceptual Models for Nursing Practice*, 3rd edn (pp. 359–68). Norwalk, Connecticut: Appleton & Lange.

Foster, P. C. and Janssens, N. P. 1980. Dorothea E. Orem. In The Nursing Theories Conference Group (eds), *Nursing theories: the base for professional nursing practice*. Englewood Cliffs, NJ: Prentice Hall.

Hanucharurnkul, S. 1989. Comparative analysis of Orem's and King's theories. *Journal of Advanced Nursing* **14**(5), 365–72.

Johnston, R. L. 1983. Orem self-care model of nursing. In Fitzpatrick, J. and Whall, A. L. (eds), *Conceptual Models of Nursing: analysis and application*. Bowie, Maryland: Robert J. Brady.

Joseph, L. S. 1980. Self-care and the nursing process. *Nursing Clinics of North America* 15(1), 131–43.

King, C. 1980. The self-care, self-help concept. *Nurse Practitioner* 5, 34–5.

Kinlein, M. L. 1977. Self-care concept. *American Journal of Nursing* 77, 598–601.

Lundh, U., Soder, M., and Waerness, K. 1988. Nursing theories: a critical view. *Image: Journal of Nursing Scholarship* 20(1), 36–40.

McFarlane, E. A. 1980. Nursing theory: the comparison of four theoretical proposals. *Journal of Advanced Nursing* 5, 3–9.

*Melnyk, K. A. M. 1983. The process of theory analysis: an examination of the nursing theory of Dorothea E. Orem. *Nursing Research* 32(3), 170–4.

Orem, D. E. 1959. *Guides for Developing Curriculae for the Education of Practical Nurses*. Washington, D.C.: US Department of Health, Education and Welfare, Office of Education.

Orem, D. E. 1971. *Nursing: Concepts of Practice*. New York: McGraw-Hill.

Orem, D. E. 1980. *Nursing: Concepts of Practice*, 2nd edn. New York: McGraw-Hill.

Orem, D. E. 1983. The self-care deficit theory of nursing: a general theory. In Clements, I. W., and Roberts, F. B. (eds), *Family Health: a theoretical approach to nursing care*, pp. 205–17. New York: Wiley.

*Orem, D. E. 1985. *Nursing: Concepts of Practice*, 3rd edn. New York: McGraw-Hill.

*Orem, D. E. 1991. *Nursing: Concepts of Practice*, 4th edn. New York: McGraw-Hill.

Orem, D. E. and Taylor, S. G. 1986. Orem's general theory of nursing. In Winstead-Fry, P. (ed.), *Case Studies in Nursing Theory*. New York: National League for Nursing.

Riehl-Sisca, J. 1989. Orem's general theory of nursing: an interpretation. In *Conceptual Models for Nursing Practice*, 3rd edn (pp.369–75). Norwalk, Connecticut: Appleton & Lange.

Rosenbaum, J. N. 1986. Comparison of two theorists on care: Orem and Leininger. *Journal of Advanced Nursing* 11(4), 409–19.

Runtz, S. E. and Urtel, J. G. 1983. Evaluating your practice via a nursing model ... the Orem self-care model and the Peplau interpersonal process model. *Nurse Practitioner: American Journal of Primary Health Care* 3(3), 30, 32, 37–40.

Silva, M. C. 1986. Research testing nursing theory: state of the art. *Advances in Nursing Science* 9(1), 1–11.

Smith, M. C. 1979. Proposed metaparadigm for nursing research and theory development: an analysis of Orem's self-care theory. *Image* 11(3), 75–9.

Sullivan, T. J. 1980. Self-care model for nursing. In *New Directions for Nursing in the '80s*. Kansas City: American Nurses Association.

Thibodeau, J. 1983. *Nursing Models: analysis and evaluation*. California: Wadsworth.

Uys, L. R. 1987. Foundational studies in nursing ... Orem, King and Rogers. *Journal of Advanced Nursing* 12(3), 275–80.

143

*Walker, L. and Avant, K. 1983. *Strategies for Theory Construction in Nursing*. Norwalk, Connecticut: Appleton-Century-Crofts.

Walton, J. 1985. An overview: Orem's self-care deficit theory of nursing. *Focus on Critical Care* 12(1), 54–8.

Whelan, E. G. 1984. Analysis and application of Dorothea Orem's self-care practice model. *Journal of Nursing Education* 23(8), 342–5.

Research

Alexander, J. S., Younger, R. E., Cohen, R. M. and Crawford, L. V. 1988. Effectiveness of a nurse-managed program for children with chronic asthma. *Journal of Pediatric Nursing: Nursing Care of Children and Families* 3(5), 312–17.

Bottorff, J. L. 1988. Assessing an instrument in a pilot project: the self-care agency questionnaire. *Canadian Journal of Nursing Research* 20(1), 7–16.

Chang, B. L. 1980. Evaluation of heath care professionals in facilitating self-care: review of the literature and a conceptual model. *Advances in Nursing Science* 3(1), 43–58.

Clinton, J., Denyes, M., Goodwin, J. and Koto, E. 1979. Developing criterion measures of nursing care: case study of a process. *Journal of Nursing Administration* 7, 41–5.

Coward, D. D. 1988. Hypercalcemia knowledge assessment in patients at risk of developing cancer-induced hypercalcemia. *Oncology Nursing Forum* 15(4), 471–6.

Denyes, M. J. 1982. Measurement of self-care agency in adolescents (abstract). *Nursing Research* 31, 63.

Denyes, M. J. 1988. Orem's model used for health promotion: directions from research. *Advances in Nursing Science* 11(1), 13–21.

Ewing, G. 1989. The nursing preparation of stoma patients for self-care. *Journal of Advanced Nursing* 14(5), 411–20.

Fernsler, J. 1986. A comparison of patient and nurse perceptions of patients' self-care deficits associated with cancer chemotherapy. *Cancer Nursing* 9(2), 50–7.

Geden, E. 1989. The relationship between self-care theory and empirical research. In Riehl-Sisca, J. (ed.), *Conceptual Models for Nursing Practice*, 3rd edn (pp. 377–82). Norwalk, Connecticut: Appleton & Lange.

Green, L. W. *et al.* 1977. Research and demonstration issues in self-care: measuring the decline of medicocentricism. *Health Education Monographs* 5, 161–81.

Hanucharurnkul, S. 1989. Predictors of self-care in cancer patients receiving radiotherapy. *Cancer Nursing* 12(1), 21–7.

Harper, D. C. 1984. Application of Orem's theoretical constructs to self-care medication behaviors in the elderly. *Advances in Nursing Science* 6(3), 29–46.

Hartley, L. A. 1988. Congruence between teaching and learning self-care: a pilot study. *Nursing Science Quarterly* 1(4), 161–7.

Hartweg, D. L. and Metcalfe, S. A. 1986. Self-care attitude changes of nursing students enrolled in a self-care curriculum – a longitudinal study. *Research in Nursing & Health* 9(4), 347–53.

Harvey, B. L. 1988. Self-care practices to prevent low back pain. *AAOHN Journal* 36(5), 211–17, 246–8.

Hayward, M. B., Kish, J. P., Jr., Frey, G. M., Kirchner, J. M., Carr, L. S. and Wolfe, C. M. 1989. An instrument to identify stressors in renal transplant recipients. *ANNA Journal* 16(2), 81–4.

*Kearney, B. Y. and Fleischer, B. J. 1979. Development of an instrument to measure exercise of self-care agency. *Research in Nursing and Health* 2(1), 25–34.

*Kuriansky, J., Gurland, B., Fleiss, J., and Cowan, D. 1976. The assessment of self-care capacity in geriatric psychiatric patients by objective and subjective methods. *Journal of Clinical Psychology* 32, 95–102.

*McBride, S. 1987. Validation of an instrument to measure exercise of self-care agency. *Research in Nursing & Health* 10(5), 311–16.

Rhodes, V. A., Watson, P. M. and Hanson, B. M. 1988. Patient's descriptions of the influence of tiredness and weakness on self-care abilities. *Cancer Nursing* 11(3), 186–94.

Sandman, P. O., Norberg, A., Adolfsson, R., Axelsson, K. and Hedly, V. 1986. Nursing care of patients with Alzheimer-type dementia: a theoretic model based on direct observations. *Journal of Advanced Nursing* 11(4), 369–78.

Schafer, S. L. 1989. An aggressive approach to promoting health responsibility. *Journal of Gerontological Nursing* 15(4), 22–7, 40–1.

Whall, A. L. 1987. Self-care responses to respiratory illnesses among Vietnamese. *Western Journal of Nursing Research* 9(2), 237–9.

Woodtli, A. O. 1988. Changes in the exercise of self-care agency. *Western Journal of Nursing Research* 10(3), 269–71.

Youssef, F. A. 1987. Discharge planning for psychiatric patients: the effects of a family-patient teaching programme. *Journal of Advanced Nursing* 12(5), 611–16.

Practice

Allison, S. E. 1973. A framework for nursing action in a nurse-conducted diabetic management clinic. *Journal of Nursing Administration* 3(4), 53–60.

Anna, D. J., Christensen, D. G., Hohon, S. A. and Wells, S. R. 1978. Implementing Orem's conceptual framework. *Journal of Nursing Administration* 8(1), 8–11.

*Backscheider, J. E. 1974. Self-care requirement, self-care capabilities, and nursing systems in the diabetic nurse management clinic. *American Journal of Public Health* 64, 1138–46.

Behi, R. 1986. Look after yourself ... Orem's self-care model. *Nursing Times* 82(37), 35–7.

Bower, F. N. and Patterson, J. 1986. A theory-based nursing assessment of the aged ... Orem's self-care model. *Topics in Clinical Nursing* 8(1), 22–32.

Bromley, B. 1980. Applying Orem's self-care theory in interostomal therapy. *American Journal of Nursing* 80, 245–9.

Buckwalter, K. C. and Kerfoot, K. M. 1982. Teaching patients self-care: a critical aspect of psychiatric discharge planning. *Journal of Psychiatric Nursing and Mental Health Services* 20(5), 299–305.

Cammermeyer, M. 1983. Growth model of self-care for neurologically impaired people. *Journal of Neurosurgical Nursing* 15, 299–305.

Campuzano, M. 1982. Self-care following coronary artery bypass surgery. *Focus* (April-May), 55–6.

Chavasse, J. 1988. A tailor-made course: curriculum planning in miniature. *Nurse Education Today* 8(4), 222–8.

Cheetham, T. 1988. Model care in the surgical ward ... adapting Orem's model in paediatrics. *Senior Nurse* 8(4), 10–12.

Clark, M. D. 1986. Application of Orem's theory of self-care: a case study. *Journal of Community Health Nursing* 3(3), 127–35.

Coleman, L. J. 1980. Orem's self-care concept of nursing. In Riehl, J. P. and Roy, C. (eds), *Conceptual Models for Nursing Practice*, 2nd edn (pp. 314–28). New York: Appleton-Century-Crofts.

Compton, P. 1989. Drug abuse: a self-care deficit. *Journal of Psychosocial Nursing and Mental Health Services* 27(3), 22–6.

*Dashiff, C. J. 1988. Theory development in psychiatric-mental health nursing: an analysis of Orem's theory. *Archives of Psychiatric Nursing* 2(6), 366–72.

*De la Cruz, L. A. D. 1988. In search of psychiatric nursing theory: an exploration of Orem's self-care model's applicability. *Canadian Journal of Psychiatric Nursing* 29(3), 10–16.

Denyes, M. J., O'Connor, N. A., Oakley, D. and Ferguson, S. 1989. Integrating nursing theory, practice and research through collaborative research. *Journal of Advanced Nursing* 14(2), 141–5.

Dropkin, M. J. 1981. Development of a self-care teaching program for postoperative head and neck patients. *Cancer Nursing* (April), 29–40.

Facteau, L. 1980. Self-care concepts and the care of the hospitalized child. *Nursing Clinics of North America* 15, 145–55.

Field, P. A. 1987. The impact of nursing theory on the clinical decision making process. *Journal of Advanced Nursing* 12(5), 563–71.

Fields, L. M. 1987. A clinical application of the Orem nursing model in labor and delivery. *Emphasis: Nursing* 2(2), 102–8.

Fitzgerald, S. 1980. Utilizing Orem's self-care nursing model in designing an educational program for the diabetic. *Topics in Clinical Nursing* 2(2), 57–65.

Greenfield, E. and Pace, J. C. 1985. Orem's self-care theory of nursing: practical application to the end stage renal disease (ESRD) patient. *Journal of Nephrology Nursing* 2(4), 187–93.

Gulick, E. E. 1989. Model confirmation of the MS-related symptom checklist. *Nursing Research* **38**(3), 147–53.

Hankes, D. 1984. Self-care: assessing the aged client's need for independence. *Journal of Gerontological Nursing* **10**, 27–31.

Harris, J. 1980. Self-care is possible after caesarean delivery. *Nursing Clinics of North America* **15**, 191–4.

Herrington, J. V. and Houston, S. 1984. Using Orem's theory: a plan for all seasons. *Nursing & Health Care* **5**(1), 45–7.

Hill, L. and Smith, N. 1985. *Self-Care Nursing*. Englewood Cliffs, NJ: Prentice-Hall.

Hicks, S. 1987. The nurse and the patient: partners in education. *Canadian Critical Care Nursing Journal* **4**(3), 18–22.

Horgan, P. A. 1987. Health status perceptions affect health-related behaviors. *Journal of Gerontological Nursing* **13**(2), 30–3, 34–5.

Iveson-Iveson, J. 1982. Putting ideas into action ... Orem's self care nursing model. *Nursing Mirror* **155**(16), 49.

Jones, A. 1988. A level of independence. *Nursing Times* **84**(15), 54–7.

Karl, J. F. 1982. The effect of an exercise program on self-care activities for the institutionalized elderly. *Journal of Gerontological Nursing* **8**, 282–5.

Kinlein, M. 1977. The self-care concept. *American Journal of Nursing* **77**, 598–601.

Laurie-Shaw, B. and Ives, S. M. 1988. Implementing Orem's self-care deficit theory: selecting a framework and planning for implementation (Part 1). *Canadian Journal of Nursing Administration* **1**(1), 9–12.

Laurie-Shaw, B. and Ives, S. M. 1988. Implementing Orem's self-care deficit theory: adopting a conceptual framework of nursing (Part 2). *Canadian Journal of Nursing Administration* **1**(2), 16–19.

Levin, L. 1978. Patient education and self-care. How do they differ? *Nursing Outlook* **26**(3), 170–5.

McCoy, S. 1989. Teaching self-care in a market-oriented world. *Nursing Management* **20**(5), 22, 26.

*MacLellan, M. 1989. Community care of a patient with multiple sclerosis. *Nursing (London): The Journal of Clinical Practice, Education and Management* **3**(33), 28–32.

Michos, S. M. 1985. The application of Orem's conceptual framework to enhance self-care in a dialysis program. *ANNA Journal* **12**(1), 21–4.

Miller, J. F. 1982. Categories of self-care needs of ambulatory patients with diabetes. *Journal of Advanced Nursing* **7**, 25–31.

Millio, N. 1977. Self-care in urban settings. *Health Education Monographs* **5**, 136–44.

Morse, W. and Werner, J. S. 1988. Individualization of patient care using Orem's theory. *Cancer Nursing* **11**(3), 195–202.

Moscovitz, A. O. 1984. Orem's theory as applied to psychiatric nursing. *Perspectives in Psychiatric Care* **22**(1), 36–8.

*Mulkeen, H. 1989. Diabetes: teaching the teaching of self-care. *Nursing Times* **85**(3), 63–5.

147

*Mullin, V. I. 1980. Implementing the self-care concept in the acute care setting. *Nursing Clinics of North America* 15(1), 177–90.

Murphy, P. P. 1981. The hospice model and self-care theory. *Oncology Nursing Forum* 8(2), 19–21.

Norris, C. M. 1979. Self-care. *American Journal of Nursing* 79(3), 486–9.

Penn, C. 1988. Promoting independence. *Journal of Gerontological Nursing* 14(3), 14–19, 38–40.

Porter, D. and Shamian, J. 1983. Self-care in theory and practice. *Canadian Nurse* 79(8), 21–3.

Raven, M. 1988. Application of Orem's self-care model to nursing practice in developmental disability. *Australian Journal of Advanced Nursing* 6(2), 16–19.

Roberts, C. S. 1982. Identifying the real patient problems. *Nursing Clinics of North America* 17(3), 481–9.

Romine, S. 1986. Applying Orem's theory of self-care to staff development. *Journal of Nursing Staff Development* 2(2), 77–9.

*Storm, D. S. and Baumgartner, R. G. 1987. Achieving self-care in the ventilator-dependent patient: a critical analysis of a case study. *International Journal of Nursing Studies* 24(2), 95–106.

Taylor, S. G. 1988. Nursing theory and nursing process: Orem's theory in practice. *Nursing Science Quarterly* 1(3), 11–19.

Toyama, A. K., Edlefsen, P., Krozek, K. S., Ballantyne, S., Hostrup, M. and Wuertzer, A. 1988. Assisting long-term patient recovery through nonmonitor maintenance component in a cardiac rehabilitation program. *Journal of Cardiovascular Nursing* 2(3), 13–22.

Underwood, P. R. 1980. Facilitating self-care. In Pothier, P. (ed.). *Psychiatric Nursing* (pp. 115–44). Boston: Little, Brown.

Wagnild, G., Rodriguez, W. and Pritchett, G. 1987. Orem's self-care theory: a tool for education and practice. *Journal of Nursing Education* 26(8), 342–3.

Walborn, K. A. 1980. A nursing model for hospice, primary and self-care. *Nursing Clinics of North America* 15(1), 205–17.

Walsh, M. 1989. Asthma: the Orem self-care nursing model approach. *Nursing (London): The Journal of Clinical Practice, Education and Management* 3(38), 19–21.

Weis, A. 1988. Cooperative care: an application of Orem's self-care theory. *Patient Education and Counseling* 11(2), 141–6.

Williams, A. J. 1986. Self-care model: an assessment tool based on Orem's theory. *Nursing Success Today* 3(7), 26–8.

Wise, G. 1985. Learning to live with multiple sclerosis ... Orem's nursing model. *Nursing Times* 81(15), 37–40.

Wright, J. 1988. Trolley full of trouble ... an elderly lady with an ulcerated leg. *Nursing Times* 84(9), 24–6.

Zinn, A. 1986. A self-care program for hemodialysis patients based on Dorothea Orem's concepts. *Journal of Nephrology Nursing* 3(2), 65–77.

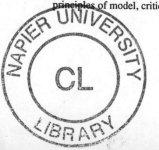

150